AIDS and Long-Term Care

A NEW DIMENSION

AIDS and Long-Term Care

A NEW DIMENSION

EDITED BY

Donna Lind Infeld, PhD
Richard McK. F. Southby, PhD, FHA

National Health Publishing

A Division of Williams & Wilkins

362,196
A28892

Published by
National Health Publishing
99 Painters Mill Road
Owings Mills, Maryland 21117
(301) 363-6400

A Division of Williams & Wilkins

Printed in the United States of America
First Printing

Designer: Sandy Renovetz
Compositor: National Health Publishing
Printer: McNaughton & Gunn

ISBN: 1-55857-009-8
LC: 89-060-360

To Marcel D. Infeld and Janet R. Southby
with our love and appreciation

CONTENTS

List of Contributors   xi
Foreword by Ben Burdetsky   xiii
Acknowledgments   xv

Introduction
Current Issues in Long-Term Care xvii
Donna Lind Infeld

Definitions of long-term care xvii   The current environment xix
The current issues xxii   AIDS patient population xxiii
Similarities among patient groups xxv   Overview xxvi
References xxvi

Part I   **Personal Impact of the Disease** 1

1. **AIDS and the Healthcare Worker** 3
Mary E. Willy and David K. Henderson

Historical perspective 3   The virus, pathogenesis, and
serological tests 4   Natural history of HIV infection 5
Epidemiology 6   Routes of transmission 7   Healthcare worker
risk 9   Prevention 16   Conclusions 19   References 19

2. **A Personal AIDS Story** 25
G.M. "Missy" LeClaire

3. **Psychosocial Issues** 31
John Maddix

Ethical issues 35   Lack of policy 36   Homophobia 37   Loss
and grief 39   Conclusions 41   References 44

Part II   **Long-Term Care Strategy and Management** 47

4. **The Need for a Long-Term Care Strategy** 49
Dennis P. Andrulis

Inpatient treatment and out-of hospital placement 50
Objectives of an AIDS long-term care system 52   System

components 52   Development of a long-term care system 55
Obstacles 57   Conclusions 57   References 58

5. **Nursing Home Care** 59
   Robert C. Marlowe

   Staff/staff family concerns 60   Patient/patient family
   concerns 62   Managerial concerns 63   Conclusions 69
   References 70

6. **Hospice Care** 71
   Monica Adams Koshuta

   Description of the hospice program 71   The hospice concept 72
   Commitment 73   Implementation 75   Conclusions 78
   References 78

7. **The Consumer's Perspective: Matching Patient Needs
   with Service Capacity** 79
   Ann Wyatt

   Barriers to long-term care in nursing homes 79   Medical appropriateness 82   The traditional role of nursing homes 83
   Targeted Services 85   Conclusions 87   References 89

8. **Ethical and Legal Concerns** 91
   Susan Harris

   Applicable law 91   Ethical considerations 93   Key issues 95
   Other issues 97   Conclusions 98   References 98

PART III   Financing AIDS Services 101

9. **National Issues** 103
   Mary Ann Baily

   The broader context 103   Underlying value questions 105
   Current financing patterns 106   Critical issues for the
   future 109   Conclusions 113   References 114

10. Focus on State Roles in Financing Options 115

Richard E. Merritt

The current state financing system 115   Options for states 117
The role of Medicaid 119   Indigent care programs 123
Programs for target populations 124   Assuring access 125
Conclusions 125   References 126

PART IV   Issues of Public Policy 127

11. Provider Perspective: A Double Dilemma 129

L. Gregory Pawlson and Lois A. Wiechmann

Current policies and patterns 131   Toward an optimal
solution 135   What is likely to be 136   Conclusions 137
References 138

12. The Policy Analyst's Perspective 141

Ruth S. Hanft

HIV patient characteristics 142   Financing acute HIV care 143
Long-term care 145   Costs of care 146   Ethical issues 147
Conclusions 148   References 148

13. The Public Health Perspective 151

Reed V. Tuckson

The public policy process 151   Models of care arrangements 152   Organization and management 155
Conclusions 155

14. The Federal Perspective 157

Robert E. Windom

Intragovernmental Task Force on AIDS Health Care
Delivery 158   Conclusions 161   References 161

Epilogue
A Call for Action 163
   Donna Lind Infeld and Richard McK. F. Southby
   Nursing homes 163   Issues and questions for consideration 165

Index   167

Dennis P. Andrulis, Ph.D., Vice President for Research and Policy, National Association of Public Hospitals, Washington, D.C.

Mary Ann Baily, Ph.D., Associate Research Professor of Economics and Health Care Sciences, The George Washington University, Washington, D.C.

Ruth S. Hanft, M.A., Research Professor, Department of Health Services Administration, The George Washington University, Washington, D.C.

Susan Harris, R.N., J.D., General Counsel, American Health Care Association, Washington, D.C.

David K. Henderson, M.D., Hospital Epidemiologist, Warren Grant Magnuson Clinical Center, National Institutes of Health, Bethesda, Maryland

Donna Lind Infeld, Ph.D., Associate Professor, Department of Health Services Administration, The George Washington University, Washington, D.C.

Monica Adams Koshuta, M.S.N., R.N., Administrator, The Hospice of Washington, Washington, D.C.

G.M. "Missy" LeClaire, Widow and caregiver, Washington, D.C.

John Maddix, M.S.W., Coordinator of Training, Whitman-Walker Clinic, Washington, D.C.

Robert C. Marlowe, M.B.A., President, Health Facilities Management, Inc., New Port Ritchie, Florida

Richard E. Merritt, M.A., M.A.L.D., Director, Intergovernmental Health Policy Project, Washington, D.C.

L. Gregory Pawlson, M.D., M.P.H., Acting Chairman and Professor of Health Care Sciences, Medicine, and Health Services Administration, The George Washington University, Washington, D.C.

Richard McK. F. Southby, Ph.D., Chairman and Gordon A Friesen, Professor of Health Services Administration, Department of Health Services Administration, and Professor of Health Care Sciences, The George Washington University, Washington, D.C.

Reed V. Tuckson, M.D., Commissioner of Public Health, Government of the District of Columbia

Lois A. Wiechmann, M.S., Educational Coordinator, Department of Health Care Sciences, The George Washington University, Washington, D.C.

Mary E. Willy, B.S.N., M.P.H., Infection Control Specialist, Warren Grant Magnuson Clinical Center, National Institutes of Health, Bethesda, Maryland

Robert E. Windom, M.D., Assistant Secretary, Department of Health and Human Services, Washington, D.C.

Ann Wyatt, National Citizens' Coalition for Nursing Home Reform, Washington, D.C.

The chapters in this book are based on presentations at the Fourth Annual Harold and Jane Hirsh Symposium held at The George Washington University on January 21 and 22, 1988. The chapters are clearly more than the verbal presentations; they reflect extensive revisions and updating of the materials presented at the symposium.

I believe that this book indicates that the prime objectives of the Hirsh Symposium were achieved. First, a distinguished group of citizens was assembled to discuss an important current health policy issue; and second, the content of the presentations has been produced as a book for wider public dissemination. There is no doubt that AIDS is of tremendous public health significance, not only in the United States but throughout the world. Its significance is likely to increase, rather than diminish, in the immediate future. Until this symposium was held, there was scant attention paid to the relationship between this disease and long-term care. This book clearly underlines the extent and significance of this relationship.

Ben Burdetsky, Ph.D.
Acting Dean
School of Government and Business Administration
The George Washington University

——— A C K N O W L E D G M E N T S ———

The University is grateful to Dr. and Mrs. Harold Hirsh for their generous annual grants which make these symposia possible. We hope that these programs will continue as important contributions to the health policy debates in this country in the future.

In addition to all the contributors and participants in the 1988 symposium, we would like to express our gratitude to Mr. Syed Hossain, Senior Word Processing Operator, and Ms. Colleen Sonosky, Office Supervisor, in the Department of Health Services Administration, for their exceptional contributions to the production of this book.

INTRODUCTION

Current Issues in
Long-Term Care

Donna Lind Infeld

This is a time of change in long-term care delivery especially in the areas of financing mechanisms and quality assurance procedures. In addition, challenging new populations have arisen, including ventilator-dependent patients, chronically ill children, and perhaps of most critical concern, persons with acquired immunodeficiency syndrome (AIDS) and others who carry the human immunodeficiency virus (HIV-1). Our goal is to set the framework for examining the impact of patients with AIDS and with AIDS-related complex (ARC) on long-term care, including issues of management, finance, ethics and law, and public policy.

Before examining these new areas, it is important to have a clear understanding of existing conditions in the long-term care arena. Only then will it be possible to move on to an examination of both the long-term care needs of AIDS patients and the availability of services to meet those needs. Finally, this book will examine policy questions and conclude with recommendations for future research and policy directions.

This book cannot answer all of the questions it poses. However, our hope is that it will stimulate further research and action on a problem which has fallen through the cracks in most discussions including the provision of health care to people with AIDS, namely, the issue of long-term care.

There has been considerable debate regarding the scope of these discussions. Should the concern be focused only on people with AIDS (PWAs)? Should it also include those with ARC (a group of relatively minor, chronic debilitating symptoms including diarrhea, weight loss, fever, etc.)? Broader yet, should it include all persons with HIV infection (most of whom are asymptomatic) as the population of concern? Since some of the manifestations of disease related to the HIV virus are still emerging, the term *HIV-related disorders* or *disease* will be used to include all those with health problems related to HIV infection, and the term *AIDS* will refer specifically to those persons having the disease manifestation defined as AIDS by the Centers for Disease Control (CDC). Since HIV-1 is the predominant form of the human immunodeficiency virus in the United States, HIV will be used hereinafter to refer specifically to HIV-1.

This book deals with the problems created by the presence of patients with HIV. However, we also recognize that the diagnosis of AIDS or ARC may be the only way to know that a patient carries the virus, and further, that such a diagnosis may directly affect which services are reimbursable by public or private sources. Therefore, even in a broad focus of providing care to anyone with HIV infection, specific attention to those diagnosed with AIDS or ARC is warranted.

Definitions of Long-Term Care

Although there are many definitions of long-term care, several of those used most often follow.

Long-term care is "directed at providing continuing care for the functionally impaired in the least restrictive environment; long-term care sits uncomfortably on the boundary between health and social services and includes elements of both" (Kane and Kane 1987, 3).

"Long-term care is a set of health, personal care, and social services delivered over a sustained period of time to persons who have lost or never acquired some degree of functional capacity" (Kane and Kane 1987, 4).

"Long-term care consists of those services designed to provide diagnostic, preventative, therapeutic, rehabilitative, supportive, and maintenance services for individuals of all age groups who have chronic physical and/or mental impairments, in a variety of institutional and noninstitutional health care settings, including the home, with the goal of promoting the optimum level of physical, social, and psychological functioning" (Koff 1982, 3).

These definitions share two features. First, they emphasize the functional capacity of individuals rather than diagnosis, age, or any specific setting. Second, and of primary concern here, they all would include AIDS patients.

The Current Environment

The Population

A wide range of estimates exist as to how many people need long-term care. One such estimate indicates that there are 6.4 million people who require the help of another person in order to carry on everyday activities. Of these people, 4.9 million live in the community, and 1.5 million live in nursing homes (Oriol 1985).

Approximately 1.2 million elderly residents live in 26,000 nursing homes. Their primary diagnoses include diseases of the circulatory system, mental disorders, diabetes, and arthritis (Rabin and Stockton 1987). An additional 2.8 million elderly persons need assistance in the community (Oriol 1985). Besides them, approximately 900,000 chronically mentally ill patients are institutionalized, of whom 750,000 are in nursing homes (Oriol 1985).

The developmentally disabled population includes about 3.9 million people with cerebral palsy, autism, mental retardation, and other severely disabling conditions (Oriol 1985). Quadripligia, brain injuries, and other physical handicaps cause people of all ages to need long-term care. The data on the prevalence of these conditions are very limited, but the numbers seem to be increasing. Finally, the population of disabled infants and chronically ill children also appears to be increasing, perhaps in part due to the growing survival rate of premature infants with major chronic conditions (Hughes 1986).

The Service Systems

Even though the types of services required by these various populations are similar, they tend to be provided by different service systems. To a large extent, this has been caused by the separate funding sources for each condition or diagnosis. Despite these distinctions, there is substantial overlap in certain settings, most

notably in nursing homes. This is due in part to a growing population with multiple long-term care needs, e.g., the elderly mentally
retarded and the elderly mentally ill. Paradoxically, there is also a
shortage of services, making it difficult to provide the most appropriate setting for all who need care.

Many efforts have been made to coordinate the delivery of long-
term care into a system or, more precisely, into several separate
systems, one for each population group. These efforts have had
some limited success. In most communities, however, locating long-
term care is an enormously difficult task for members of any of the
population groups. It appears to be even worse for people with
AIDS.

Some of the service settings in these various long-term care
systems have particular applicability to people with AIDS. Nursing
homes are the most visible component of long-term care. The nursing home industry is characterized by small, primarily proprietary
facilities, increasingly owned by large chains and operating at near
full capacity. Ninety percent of nursing home patients are over the
age of 65 (Oriol 1985).

Skilled nursing facilities provide continuous nursing care to
patients who require rehabilitation or skilled nursing care on an
inpatient basis. Intermediate care patients, on the other hand, do not
require continuous skilled nursing care. They may be ambulatory or
nonambulatory and require some level of monitoring and ongoing
assistance with daily activities (Intergovernmental Health Policy
Project 1987, 7–14). Few AIDS patients are cared for in nursing
homes. The reasons for this lack of utilization are discussed in later
chapters of this book (see the chapters by Andrulis, Marlowe, and
Wyatt in particular).

Residential care facilities provide nonmedical care in settings
such as board and care homes, domiciliary or group homes. These
facilities provide housing, meals, supervision, and assistance with
daily activities such as eating, bathing, dressing, toileting, and
taking medications. Only in a very few locations are these facilities
available to people with AIDS. One example of this type of facility
was described in the *Washington Post* on January 18, 1988 (Colburn).
This new facility will serve as a community home for four children
under the age of 6 years old who have AIDS.

Hospices have been the organizations most willing to respond to the needs of AIDS patients. However, even here, the question arises of whether there should be separate hospices providing care to AIDS patients or whether all hospices should share in this responsibility.

Other services are provided in community-based settings such as clinics, community centers, and day care facilities, enabling patients to maintain a household while receiving services in a group setting. In some high prevalence areas such as San Francisco and New York City, networks of community-based services have developed specifically for people with AIDS. The questions remains as to what can be done in lower prevalence areas.

Adult day care programs offer protective settings providing a range of health and/or social services on a less than 24 hour per day basis. Adult day care programs are located in hospitals, nursing homes, social service agencies, or they may be freestanding. Most often they are small and nonprofit, and most operate under capacity because they lack third party funding. The problem of lack of access occurs for both geriatric and AIDS patients, although it is more extreme in the latter group. Is it feasible for one adult day care program to provide care for people with AIDS as well as for the elderly? If feasible, would this be desirable?

Home care involves providing in the home setting preventive, supportive, rehabilitative, or therapeutic health care which may include skilled nursing, chore assistance, personal and social work services. These services enable patients to remain in their homes while receiving ongoing medical monitoring. Increasingly, specialized home medical services are evolving to meet the maintenance needs of AIDS patients, but there are serious problems of reimbursement. Less than a quarter of hospital-based home care programs currently provide care to AIDS patients due in part to limited funding (Intergovernmental Health Policy Project 1987).

Respite care is primarily designed to relieve the burden of care on family members or to provide it when those caretakers are at work or otherwise unavailable. Respite care is also in very short supply. Questions similar to those of concern in home care and community-based services also face respite care: Who should provide the care? Where? For whom? How should it be paid for?

Coordination is central to the successful delivery of both home care and community-based care. Case management programs (more recently referred to as service management) usually involve a nurse or social worker providing assessment and monitoring of the provision of multiple services. Service management programs are available for the general long-term care population in some urban areas. These services are available in even fewer communities for AIDS patients.

The Current Issues

Despite the existence of this variety of long-term care services there are several areas of current concern. Chief among them are the quality of care, access to care, cost, and reimbursement.

Quality

Long-term care is primarily a minimum wage industry with the greatest amount of direct patient contact coming from nursing aides. As a result, there are ongoing problems of staff shortages and chronic high turnover rates. In addition, there are difficulties measuring and monitoring the quality of care, especially in home-delivered services.

Access

Nursing homes are generally full and often have lengthy waiting lists. Some reimbursement systems encourage priority admission of light care rather than heavy care patients, making it particularly difficult for very sick persons, especially those on Medicaid, to locate care. Home health and community services are in limited supply and are typically short on funding. Fear of increasing public costs has resulted in efforts to contain the supply of services (especially nursing home beds) and to focus on screening programs to assure appropriate placements.

Cost

Nursing homes are very expensive, and few patients have insurance coverage for them. While community-based alternatives may be less expensive on a per patient basis, on a system-wide basis they cost more because of greater demand. AIDS patients may find long-term care to be a low cost option compared with hospitalization, but AIDS patients are a high cost group for the long-term care settings to serve.

Reimbursement

Medicaid is the primary payor of nursing home care, and states have a range of reimbursement strategies which influence the types of patients most likely to receive care. A growing number of states are moving toward case-mix reimbursement under Medicaid, creating an incentive for the nursing home to take sicker patients, and thereby potentially improving access for AIDS patients. These programs, however, are still in the minority.

AIDS Patient Population

It is important to remember that there is not one AIDS population; there are at least three, each of which has unique long-term care needs.

Gay Males

Although this group is now the largest among AIDS patients, it is projected to peak in the next several years and then decrease as other population groups grow.

Children

The Intergovernmental Health Policy Project report states that:

In general, the difficulties of caring for terminal patients are exacerbated when caring for children with AIDS. The majority of pediatric cases come from low income families who lack the financial and social resources needed to provide even minimal care. When one or both parents use drugs, the problems are magnified because resources are frequently limited and undependable (Intergovernmental Health Policy Project 1987, 7–8).

Even states with high incidence and specialized programs primarily depend on hospital-based programs with supportive home services to care for children with AIDS. There is a serious problem of abandoned children who presently tend to stay in the hospital. Estimates are that by 1991 there will be more than six times the number of infants and children with AIDS and few services available for their care (Intergovernmental Health Policy Project 1987).

Intravenous Drug Users

This subgroup of the AIDS population is projected to increase (Jenna 1987). Drug users have special problems and are hard to reach. The group includes a high proportion of minorities who may need other support services such as housing, and who often have medical complications related to poor health and nutrition (Institute of Medicine 1986). An additional concern is that the increasing AIDS prevalence among drug users will likely result in more heterosexual and pediatric AIDS patients.

Other Groups

Smaller AIDS population groups include elderly men and women who may have received infected blood transfusions, and women who have received the virus from a sexual partner.

In addition to being separate populations based on age, lifestyle, and support systems, there are also distinct populations in terms of clinical needs.

Neurological Complications

One group of patients who pose special problems is that of persons suffering from neurological complications. Patients infected with HIV have a high incidence of central nervous system disease, sometimes resulting in severe dementia. In those instances, continuous custodial care may be required for a period of several months (Institute of Medicine 1986).

Irrespective of the level of family or social support, these patients can almost never receive adequate care in a commu-

nity-based setting, because they require 24 hour a day surveillance. Because extended care facilities, in almost all cases,
refuse admittance to patients with AIDS, dementia will lead
to extended use of acute care hospital beds unless alternatives are found (Institute of Medicine 1986, 147).

The reason for identifying these various subpopulations at the
outset of discussing AIDS and long-term care is to emphasize that
long-term care services and systems must be responsive to very
complex needs. No one service model will be appropriate for all
AIDS and ARC patients.

Similarities among Patient Groups

People with AIDS have medical needs that are very similar to
those of patients suffering from other chronic illnesses. According
to the Intergovernmental Health Policy Project, 1987, they require:
consistent on-going care; self-management and monitoring to prevent rapid escalation of infections; and immediate treatment to
prevent debilitation when infections occur (Rowe and Ryan 1987).
Also, like other long-term care, AIDS care is nurse-centered rather
than focusing on physician treatments (Jenna 1987).

Despite these similarities, however, AIDS and ARC patients are
more difficult to serve than other chronic care patients for several
reasons.

1. The staff members do not have enough training and
   tend to have high levels of anxiety and fear.

2. AIDS patients need a great deal of skilled care including
   extensive emotional support.

3. Medical monitoring is needed to prevent recurrent hos-
   pitalizations.

4. Varied levels of care are required intermittently.

5. Inappropriate and insufficient housing is often a barrier
   to home care.

6. AIDS patients lack knowledge of available services.

Only in a few high-risk urban areas, e.g., San Francisco, is the necessary array of services and providers designed to overcome these barriers being offered in a comprehensive manner.

Overview

The remaining chapters in this book address these many issues in greater depth. Part I includes discussion of the personal aspects of AIDS, including the impact it has had on healthcare workers, family members, and the AIDS patients themselves.

After introducing the need for a long-term care strategy for AIDS patients, Part II examines its implications for the management of nursing homes, home health care, and the hospice. The importance of matching patient needs with care settings is discussed from the perspective of a consumer group representative. Finally, ethical and legal issues among public policy providers are discussed including an examination of AIDS as a handicap, antidiscrimination laws, and the ethical basis for decisions about whom to serve.

Part III reviews the financing of AIDS services from both federal and state perspectives. Special attention is focused on new funding strategies being used at the state level.

Part IV looks at public policy issues from four different viewpoints: the provider, the policy analyst, local public health organizations, and the federal government. Topics include who pays for care, whether public support should be based on a means test, the segregation of care for AIDS patients, and issues of care rationing.

In conclusion, the epilogue is a call for expanded research efforts and the development of a continuum of care for services to meet the full range of needs presented by the crisis of AIDS.

References

Colburn, D. 1988. Children, AIDS and a special home. *The Washington Post*, 19 Jan. Health, p. 6.

Hughes, S. 1986. *Long-term care: Options in an expanding market*. Homewood, IL: Dow Jones-Irwin

Institute of Medicine. 1986. Care of persons infected with HIV. *In Confronting AIDS: Directions for Public Health, Health Care, and Research*, 139–173. Washington, D.C.: National Academy Press

Jenna, J.K. 1987. AIDS management: New models for care. *Healthcare Forum Journal* Nov./Dec.: 18–48.

Kane, R.A., and R.L. Kane. 1987. *Long-term care: Principles, programs, and policies.* New York: Springer Publishing Co. Inc.

Koff, T. 1982. *Long-term care: An approach to serving the frail elderly.* Boston: Little, Brown & Co. Inc.

Oriol, W. 1985. *The complex cube of long-term care: The case for next-step solutions—now.* Washington, D.C.: American Health Planning Association.

Rabin, D.L., and P. Stockton. 1987. *Long-term care for the elderly: A factbook.* New York: Oxford University Press Inc.

Rowe, M., and C. Ryan. 1987. *AIDS: A public health challenge. Vol. 2, Managing and financing the problem,* ed. Committee on the National Strategy for AIDS. Washington, D.C.: Intergovernmental Health Policy Project.

PART I

Personal Impact
of the Disease

CHAPTER 1

AIDS and the Healthcare Worker

Mary E. Willy and David K. Henderson

Since the early 1980s, healthcare providers in many hospitals have been treating patients who have been infected with human immunodeficiency virus (HIV-1). The healthcare workers involved in the care of these patients have expressed concern about their risks for becoming infected with this virus. Worker anxiety has, at times, immobilized nursing units and added to many patients' emotional difficulties. Much of this worker anxiety can be alleviated with a review of the relevant facts about HIV regarding both the transmission as well as the risks for the healthcare worker. The purpose of this review is to provide an historical perspective, some background about HIV, current epidemiology, a summary of studies of risk among healthcare workers, and ways in which all workers can minimize their risk of infection.

Historical Perspective

The first report of what is now recognized as acquired immunodeficiency syndrome (AIDS) appeared in the June 1981 issue of the *Morbidity and Mortality Weekly Report*. This report described the unusual appearance of an opportunistic infection (*Pneumocystis carinii* pneumonia, PCP) in five male homosexuals who were not known to be immunocompromised (Centers for Disease Control 1981). Not long after this report appeared, the medical community recognized a new syndrome, occurring primarily in homosexual men, that was associated with severe immunosuppression. This syndrome was called AIDS and was soon identified as occurring in other populations, as well.

Since these early studies, patients with AIDS have been studied aggressively in an attempt to understand every aspect of the disease. In 1984, the causative agent for the new syndrome, a retrovirus, was identified. Although the virus was given several candidate names, it is now called HIV-1 (Barré-Sinoussi et al. 1983; Gallo et al. 1984) referred to here as HIV. In 1985, a blood test was approved to allow testing of blood donors for this new infection so that the blood supply might be protected (Centers for Disease Control 1985a). In 1986, the first antiretroviral agent, azidothymidine (AZT), was approved by the FDA for use in the treatment of AIDS, and that same year trials were begun at several centers to test a newly developed vaccine. In a short time span, these and other discoveries have improved the quality of life for those already infected with HIV in addition to assisting in the prevention of infection for individuals at risk.

The Virus, Pathogenesis, and Serological Tests

HIV is an RNA retrovirus which attacks T4 lymphocytes or helper cells as well as macrophages. The virus enters these cells, and the viral RNA is transcribed to DNA by an enzyme (reverse transcriptase). This proviral DNA will either insert itself into the cellular DNA, thus beginning a latent phase, or will replicate and leave the cell, destroying it as viral progeny bind from the surface (Fauci 1988).

The screening test licensed in 1985 to help identify persons infected with this virus is an enzyme-linked immunosorbent assay (ELISA) using disrupted whole virus as the antigen that checks for the presence of antibodies directed against viral proteins. Positive ELISAs are usually confirmed with a second, more specific, test called the Western blot. Use of this two-step process is important because of the possibility of false-positive ELISAs. The current ELISA tests are 99% sensitive and 99% specific under optimal laboratory conditions. Combining this highly sensitive and specific test with Western blot confirmation, there is a low probability of a false-positive testing sequence (Centers for Disease Control 1987b).

More sensitive screening tests are constantly being developed. The use of gene amplification, i.e., polymerase chain reaction, technology appears promising. This method may allow clinicians to detect latent virus and also to estimate the viral load a patient may be carrying at any particular time (Marx 1988).

Most persons exposed to HIV will develop antibodies within 6–12 weeks, however infected patients do not seroconvert for a prolonged period of time (up to 13–14 months) (Ranki et al. 1987). This "window period" can create a problem for clinicians who are testing their patients as part of a diagnostic workup. Repeat testing six months after the initial test may be advisable for patients who test negative, but have some reason to suspect infection.

Natural History of HIV Infection

A prolonged incubation period usually precedes the development of symptoms suggestive of AIDS. Currently, the mean incubation period from the initial infection to the development of AIDS exceeds seven years (Centers for Disease Control 1987a). Between 1 and 1.5 million asymptomatically infected individuals are estimated to be living in the United States (U.S. Public Health Service 1986). The rate at which these asymptomatic infected individuals will progress to the AIDS-related complex (ARC) or to AIDS (either defined as the development of an opportunistic infection or unusual cancer not normally seen in young adults) is unknown. In one cross-sectional study, nearly 34% of the individuals studied progressed from seropositivity to AIDS in a three-year period (Goedert et al. 1986). The San Francisco Department of Public Health Study reported recently that 31% of asymptomatic seropositive homosexual or bisexual men will develop AIDS in an 84-month period (Hessol et al. 1987).

The opportunistic infections and neoplasms one may see in a patient with AIDS are quite varied. Some are responsive to therapy, and others are difficult to treat. At least 80% of the patients who develop AIDS will ultimately acquire PCP, and PCP will be the initial opportunistic infection in 60% of these cases. Although patients may present with Kaposi's sarcoma or other neoplasms, more frequently they develop infections commonly seen in immunosuppressed hosts, such as toxoplasmosis, disseminated *Mycobacterium avium-intracellulare* infection, disseminated cytomegalovirus, her-

Table 1-1 Cases of AIDS Reported to the CDC as of December 5, 1988

Adults/Adolescents	Number of Cases	Percent of Total
Homosexual/bisexual male	48,625	62
Intravenous drug abuser	15,533	20
Homosexual male and intravenous drug abuser	5,662	7
Hemophilia/coagulation disorder	755	1
Heterosexual cases	3,442	4
Transfusion, blood components	1,982	3
Undetermined	2,546	3
	78,545	
Children		
Hemophilia/coagulation disorder	82	6
Parent with/at risk of AIDS	991	78
Transfusion, blood/components	162	13
Undetermined	43	3
	1,278	

pes simplex or herpes zoster virus infection, or cryptococcal meningitis (Glatt, Chirgivia, and Landesman 1988).

Epidemiology

Since 1981, 79,823 cases of AIDS have been reported to the Centers for Disease Control (CDC); 44,826 (56%) of those reported have died. As a result of its intensive AIDS surveillance activities, (Table 1-1) the CDC has identified several behaviors, including sex with an infected partner, needle sharing in IV substance abuse, and receipt of contaminated blood products, associated with a higher risk for HIV infection. Although the numbers of AIDS cases continues to increase, the percentage of AIDS cases in each transmission category has varied little since the surveillance program first began in 1981 (Centers for Disease Control 1988b).

The number of transfusion recipient cases is expected to begin to decrease as a result of the implementation of deferred donation, begun in March, 1983 and routine antibody testing of all blood donors, begun in March, 1988. Although rare, reports still appear of transfusion-associated HIV infection resulting from the seronegative blood from an individual in the window phase of the disease (Ward et al. 1988). The risk for transfusion-related infection is now very low.

Investigation of cases of AIDS occurring in patients with no identified risk (NIR) behaviors, i.e., the patient does not acknowledge participation in one of the conventional risk behaviors, shows no significant change in proportion over the years that the surveillance has been performed. As of September 30, 1987, 2,059 AIDS cases had been classified on the initial case report forms as being NIR. At the time of manuscript preparation, 921 (45%) of these cases were either still under investigation or had incomplete histories, i.e., the patient died before the interview, refused to be interviewed, or was lost to follow-up. Seventy-two percent of the remaining 1,138 patients were reclassified into one of the conventional transmission categories, and 3% of the remaining patients did not meet the CDC AIDS definitions. Only 281 patients (25% of those with complete investigations) could not be reclassified. Of the 281 patients who have undergone in-depth interviews a high proportion (178) report either a prior history of one or more sexually transmitted diseases or prior contact with a prostitute. Investigators of these NIR cases do not report finding any evidence that would suggest a new mode of transmission (Castro et al. 1988).

In the United States, 58% of adult AIDS cases and 24% of pediatric AIDS cases have occurred in Caucasians, whereas blacks have accounted for 26% of adult cases and 53% of pediatric cases, and Hispanics have accounted for 15% of adult cases and 23% of pediatric cases (Centers for Disease Control 1988b). Both blacks and Hispanics are disproportionately represented among the AIDS cases reported (11.6% of the general population is black and 6.5% is Hispanic). This overrepresentation of blacks and Hispanics is thought to be a result of the high prevalence of intravenous drug abuse among these minority populations in certain areas of the Untied States (Curran et al. 1988).

Routes of Transmission

Researchers have attempted to culture HIV from a variety of body fluids. Although the virus has been isolated from blood, semen, vaginal secretions, breast milk, saliva, cerebrospinal fluid, tears, urine, and alveolar fluid, current epidemiological evidence has implicated only four of these body fluids (blood, semen, vaginal secretions, and breast milk) as routes of transmission for HIV (Friedland and Klein 1987). The risk for HIV transmission associated with contaminated saliva is extremely small. This contention is supported by studies of dentists that report only one case of apparent occupational infection among those evaluated and by studies of the household contacts of AIDS patients that have failed to identify transmission among people who shared the patient's utensils and dental supplies. Insect vectors have not been incriminated in the transmission of HIV (Lifson 1988; Centers for Disease Control 1986a).

The commonly accepted routes of transmission for HIV include

1. percutaneous exposure to blood (either by transfusion of contaminated blood products, sharing of contaminated needles among intravenous drug abusers, experiencing an accidental needlestick [or other sharp injury] with a contaminated sharp object, or contaminating mucous membranes or an open wound with blood);

2. sexual exposure to infected body fluids; or

3. exposure of a child to an infected mother either transplacentally or at the time of delivery (perinatally) Friedland and Klein 1987).

Concerns about the risk of transmission from immune globulin preparations or from the hepatitis B vaccine that is prepared from pooled plasma have been laid to rest by intense study of the safety of these products. Review of the processing procedures required for both of these products as well as the epidemiological study of recipients of these preparations support the manufacturers' claims of safety. Immunoglobulin preparations go through a fractionation process that is calculated to remove 10^{15} infectious units of HIV per milliliter—far more virus than would be found in HIV-infected plasma (Centers for Disease Control 1986c). The hepatitis B vaccine undergoes a three-step process to inactivate all viruses (including hepatitis B virus [HBV] and HIV; each of these steps has been shown to be highly effective (Centers for Disease Control 1984).

There is no evidence to suggest that casual transmission of HIV is occurring. The best scientific support for this statement comes from the investigations of the household contacts of patients infected with HIV (Friedland and Klein 1987; Redfield et al. 1985; Fischl et al. 1987; Friedland et al. 1987). These studies have prospectively evaluated the household contacts of infected patients for serological evidence of infection. None of these studies have found evidence of casual transmission, i.e., only household contacts who have had sexual or perinatal exposure have evidence for infection. Friedland and his colleagues have studied 200 nonsexual household contacts of 85 patients with AIDS or ARC (Friedland et al. 1987). In this study, the household contacts were followed for a median of 35 months. For much of the study period, many of the household contacts were unaware that they had been living in the same household with an HIV-infected patient, since the patients were often asymptomatic for months before signs of illness developed. Household contacts in this study had a variety of casual exposures, including the sharing of towels, eating utensils, plates, razors, and toothbrushes. Only one household contact, a child born to a mother with AIDS, had evidence of infection (Friedland et al. 1987).

Healthcare Worker Risk

The greatest risk for exposure to HIV is through certain sexual behaviors or through the unsafe needle practices prevalent among intravenous drug abusers. Risks to the healthcare worker for occupationally acquired infection appear to be quite low. The evidence for this relatively low risk can be assessed by evaluating cases of AIDS reported to the CDC among healthcare workers, by studying the actual incidents resulting in occupational or nosocomial infection for common experiences, and by reviewing prospective studies of healthcare workers in progress at several institutions.

As of March, 1988, 2,586 (5.4%) of 47,532 cases of AIDS reported to the CDC had occurred in healthcare workers (Centers for Disease Control 1988c). The U.S. Department of Labor (DOL) estimates that 5.7% of the U.S. labor force is employed in the health professions. Thus, on the basis of this comparison, healthcare workers are not overrepresented in the population of patients reported to the CDC as having AIDS without an identifiable risk for HIV infection. Conversely, 5.3% of AIDS cases in healthcare workers reported to the CDC (135 cases) (compared with 2.8% of all other cases) cannot be classified into one of the traditional transmission categories. This difference is statistically significant (p < 0.001, chi-square). Thus, healthcare workers with AIDS are more likely to deny traditional risk factors for HIV infection. The overrepresentation of healthcare workers reporting "no identifiable risk" could be due to underreporting of risk behaviors, occupational exposures, or both (Centers for Disease Control 1988c).

Of the 135 healthcare workers classified on the initial AIDS case report forms as having no identifiable risk for infection, only 41 (30.4%) remain in the NIR group after follow-up interviews. Twenty of the 135 (14.8%) either refused to be interviewed or died before an investigative interview could be conducted; 74 (54.8%) are still under investigation (Centers for Disease Control 1988c).

Analysis has been completed of the 41 healthcare workers who remained in the NIR classification following investigative interviews. Males are overrepresented in this population (68%, with only 23% of all healthcare professionals being male). The only particular occupation overrepresented in this analysis was maintenance work (Centers for Disease Control 1988c). These data suggest that healthcare workers may underreport risk behaviors. If the overrepresentation of healthcare workers was due entirely to occupational risk, one would expect to see more women reported (since, as noted above, women comprise 77% of the healthcare work force), and one would also expect to find more workers whose jobs entail intense blood exposure.

Anecdotal reports of HIV infection in healthcare workers occurring as a result of percutaneous exposures to blood or body fluids from HIV-infected patients have clearly demonstrated that there is a risk for occupational or nosocomial transmission of this virus (Centers for Disease Control 1986b, 1987d, 1988a, 1988c; Gerberding and Henderson 1987; Centers for Disease Control 1987e; McCray 1986; Stricof and Morse 1986; *Lancet* 1984; Oskenhendler et al. 1986; Neisson-Vernant et al. 1986; Weiss et al. 1988; Ramsey, Smith, and Reinarz 1988; Gioananni et al. 1988; Henderson et al. 1988b; Michelet

Table 1-2 Healthcare Workers with Documented Seroconversions[a]

Case No.	Occupation	Type of Exposure	Source
1	Unknown	Needlestick	AIDS
2	Unknown	Needlestick	AIDS
3	Unknown	Needlestick	AIDS
4	Unknown	2 Needlesticks	AIDS/HIV-1-infected
5	Unknown	Needlestick	AIDS
6	Nurse	Needlestick	AIDS
7	Nurse	Needlestick	HIV-1-infected
8	Nurse	Needlestick	AIDS
9	Research laboratory worker	Cut with sharp object	Concentrated virus
10	Clinical laboratory worker	Cut with sharp object	AIDS
11	Nurse	Unknown	AIDS
12	Home healthcare provider	Cutaneous	AIDS
13	Unknown	Nonintact skin	AIDS
14	Phlebotomist	Mucous membranes	HIV-1-infected
15	Technologist	Nonintact skin	HIV-1-infected
16	Unknown	Needlestick	AIDS
17	Nurse	Mucous membranes	HIV-1-infected

[a]Modified from Centers for Disease Control. 1988c. Update: Acquired immunodeficiency syndrome and human immunodeficiency virus infection among healthcare workers. *Morbidity and Mortality Weekly Report* 37: 229–239.

et al. 1988). Seventeen healthcare workers have developed positive HIV antibody tests (seroconverted) following adverse exposures to HIV-infected patients (Table 1-2). These workers had negative antibody tests at the time of exposure, and almost all of them developed positive antibody tests within six months of the exposure. Many of these workers also developed an acute retroviral syndrome (fever, myalgias, mild adenopathy, and/or rash) associated with their infection. The majority of these exposures involved needlestick injuries, although five of the seroconversions resulted from exposures of blood or body fluids to nonintact skin or mucous membranes (Centers for Disease Control 1987e, 1986b; Gioananni et al. 1988). An additional seven workers have been reported as developing occupationally acquired HIV infection, but lack documented

Table 1-3 Cases of Healthcare Workers Who Have HIV-1 Infection
Without Documented Seroconversion

Case No.	Occupation	Type of Exposure	Source
1	Unknown	Puncture wound	AIDS
2	Unknown	2 Needlesticks	2 AIDS patients
3	Research laboratory worker	Nonintact skin	Concentrated virus
4	Home healthcare provider	Nonintact skin	AIDS
5	Dentist	Multiple needlesticks	Unknown
6	Technician	Multiple needlesticks and mucous membranes	Unknown
7	Laboratory worker	Needlesticks and puncture wound	Unknown

seroconversions. Four of these workers reported a percutaneous
exposure to an HIV-infected source, and the other three were
investigated and classified as probably occupationally acquired, but
without an identified source (McCray 1986; Weiss et al. 1988; Centers for Disease Control 1988a; Weiss et al. 1985; Grint and McEvoy
1985; Klein et al. 1988; Ponce deLeon, Sanchez-Mejorada, and Zaidi-
Jacobsen 1988) (Table 1-3).

Although these cases of occupational or nosocomial transmission document a risk for such transmission, these anecdotal reports
cannot give an accurate estimate of the magnitude of risk for the
healthcare worker. Prospective longitudinal studies of healthcare
workers do provide such an estimate. These studies provide both
numerators (number infected) as well as accurate denominators
(numbers experiencing adverse exposures) so that relative risk may
be estimated. They also provide descriptive data on the injuries
themselves, the body fluids associated with infection, and the amount
of time elapsed from exposure to seroconversion.

One of the largest healthcare worker studies is being conducted
by the CDC. This study recruits workers from around the United
States who have experienced an adverse exposure to the blood or
body fluids from an HIV-infected patient. As of December, 1987,

Table 1-4 Summary of Prospective Studies of Healthcare Worker Risk for Occupational Transmission of HIV-1

Author of Study	No. of Health Care Workers Studied	No. of Percutaneous Exposures Reported	No. of Seroconversions	Seroconversion Rate Per Event %
Marcus	582	582	3	0.52
Gerberding	180	224	1	0.45
Henderson	108	126	0	0
McEvoy	76	76	0	0
Kuhls	45	52	0	0
Wormser	48	48	0	0
Elmslie	115	115	0	0
Ramsey	31	31	1	0
Hernandez	58	58	0	0
Pizzocolo	77	77	0	0
Totals	1,320	1,389	5	0.36

1,176 workers had been enrolled, of whom 1,070 had at least one HIV serology performed at least 90 days post-exposure. Four of the 870 workers with parenteral exposures were seropositive, although only three of the four had seroconversions documented. One of the four was not tested until 10 months after a reported exposure, however, heterosexual transmission could not be excluded as a possible route of transmission because this individual's sexual partner was also seropositive. None of the workers reporting non-parenteral exposures seroconverted (Centers for Disease Control 1988c).

Ten longitudinal studies of healthcare workers have been published (Table 1-4) (Centers for Disease Control 1987e; Henderson et al. 1988; Marcus 1988; Gerberding et al. 1987; McEvoy et al. 1987; Kuhls et al. 1987; Wormser et al. 1988; Elmslie and O'Shaughnessy 1987; Hernandez et al. 1988; Pizzocolo et al. 1988). These studies all enroll workers who report adverse exposures to HIV-infected blood or body fluids and who are then followed prospectively. Combining the reports from these 10 studies allows one to estimate the relative risk for infection following percutaneous exposures. Five serocon-

versions have been documented following some type of percutaneous exposure in these studies for a rate of transmission of 0.36% (or
3.6 infections per 1,000 adverse exposures).

The risk for transmission of HIV following an adverse exposure
is much lower than that observed for HBV. The chance of HBV
illness following a needlestick contaminated with blood from an
HBV carrier ranges from 6 to 30% (60–300 per 1,000 adverse exposures) (Centers for Disease Control 1985b). HBV carriers present a
greater risk because of their higher virus load, and HBV carriers who
are also positive for "e" antigen typically have 100 million or more
viral particles per milliliter of blood (Centers for Disease Control
1985b). A patient infected with HIV is estimated to carry a viral load
that is significantly lower (Centers for Disease Control 1987d).

Even though an HIV infection might have a bleaker prognosis,
HBV infection can also cause serious morbidity and even death in
some cases. Every year, at least 0.1% of HBV infections are fulminant
and lead to death. Another 6–10% of the patients infected with HBV
become chronic carriers, and as such may pass the virus on to their
sexual partners or to their unborn children. These carrier patients are
also at risk for HBV-related cirrhosis or liver cancer (Robinson 1985).
The CDC reports that 500–600 healthcare workers are hospitalized
annually after developing occupationally acquired HBV infection,
and approximately 200 deaths each year result from them—12–15
due to fulminant hepatitis, 170–200 from cirrhosis, and 40–50 from
liver cancer (Department of Labor 1987). Clearly, HBV should be
recognized as a greater risk to healthcare workers than HIV. The
risks for other blood-borne infections such as non-A, non-B hepatitis, or human T-cell lymphotropic virus (HTLV-I) infection are
unknown. Health care workers need to be aware of the risks for
occupational infection from all blood-borne infections and must
make every effort to prevent transmission of them.

The healthcare workers' risk of transmission of HIV in the
absence of an adverse exposure appears to be too low to measure.
Serosurveys of healthcare workers working with HIV-infected patients have been unable to document transmission outside the
previously accepted adverse exposure categories of percutaneous,
mucous membranes, and open wounds. In three prospectives studies, 929 healthcare workers have been assessed for antibodies to HIV
(Henderson et al. 1988; Gerberding et al. 1987; Kuhls et al. 1987). No

healthcare worker in these studies was found to be seropositive unless participating in risk behaviors outside the healthcare setting.

In a cross-sectional study of dental professionals, Klein et al. (1988) studied 1,132 dentists, 131 hygienists, and 46 assistants. Study participants denied behavioral risk factors. The only dentist found to be seropositive reported treating high risk patients, working without gloves when he had breaks in his skin, and receiving several sharp injuries in the past.

Although a few anecdotal case reports suggest that HIV may be transmitted as a result of cutaneous exposure to blood (Centers for Disease Control 1987e, 1986b), the risk for transmission by this route is likely to be quite small. A study from our own hospital documents that such exposures occur commonly. Participants enrolled in an ongoing serosurvey of healthcare workers were asked to recall the frequency and type of body fluid exposures they had experienced in the previous year. This study was conducted prior to the implementation of "Universal Precautions" recommended by the CDC (Center for Disease Control 1987d). At lease one cutaneous exposure to blood or body fluids was reported by 442 of 668 respondents. What was most alarming was the report of 2,703 estimated cutaneous exposures to blood from known HIV-infected patients. Workers should have been using barriers for handling blood or body fluids from these patients, since HIV-infected patients were placed on blood and body fluid precautions. Despite these reported exposures, none of the participants was seropositive (Henderson, Fahey, and Willy 1988).

Gerberding and her colleagues also emphasized the frequency of preventable exposures. In their study, 56% of the participants failed to use adequate precautions when caring for patients with AIDS or when handling their specimens, and 63% of the participants did not follow proper precautions with ARC patients. None of these healthcare workers seroconverted during the course of this study (Gerberding et al. 1987). Subsequently one participant in this study seroconverted following an adverse exposure (Gerberding and Henderson 1987).

The serosurveys and prospective studies of healthcare workers experiencing adverse exposures emphasize the low risk associated with the care of HIV-infected patients. Clearly, the risk associated with providing care for these patients is no greater than other risks the worker tolerates as part of the job (exposures to other infectious diseases, exposures to toxic drugs and radioactivity, physical injury, etc.). Conversely, as Gerberding and others recently showed, many workers continue to take needless risks when caring for patients infected with HIV. The reasons for these behaviors are complex— lack of knowledge, shortage of barrier supplies, difficulty in changing old behaviors, or lack of an appropriate perception of the magnitude of the risk. Certain procedures can be followed to decrease the risk to the healthcare worker from all blood-borne disease without compromising the care to the patient.

Prevention

Unlike HBV infection which can be prevented with a safe and effective vaccine, the best available way to prevent occupationally acquired HIV infection is through safe healthcare practices. The U.S. Public Health Service has issued a series of recommendations to be used in all health settings (Centers for Disease Control 1987d, 1988d). These recommendations include the routine use of certain barriers when handling blood and body fluids, a recommendation which has been made by the CDC for many years (Centers for Disease Control 1985b) and which was supported by epidemiological and laboratory data regarding both HBV and HIV transmission.

The most recent CDC recommendations (Centers for Disease Control 1987d, 1988d) summarize the precautions needed in all healthcare settings (hospital, clinical, laboratory, dental clinic, pathology, operating room, dialysis, etc.) and call for healthcare workers to use what they call "Universal Precautions" when providing care. This new set of precautions was recommended for use with all patients, not just those with a known blood-borne illness, to prevent exposure to all blood-borne pathogens.

The rationale for these recommendations includes the following.

1. Relying on a serological test to identify infectious patients may give workers a false sense of security (Gerberding and Henderson 1987). These serological tests require that an HIV-infected patient produce antibodies detectable by the ELISA. During the period the patient

is in the process of seroconverting, the antibody tests will be negative, yet the patient will still be infectious (Ranki et al. 1987). In addition, a false-negative test is rare, but possible, as with any laboratory test where human or mechanical error can occur (Ward et al. 1988).

2. Even when patients may be known to be infected, they may not be properly identified to other personnel. Laboratory specimens may be unlabeled or mislabeled (Handsfield, Cummings, and Swenson 1987).

3. There are no laboratory tests commercially available to test for carriers of some blood-borne infections such as HTLV-IV and non-A, non-B hepatitis.

4. Blood-borne pathogens may exist that are as yet unknown to the medical community.

5. There are many settings within a healthcare institution where screening patients would not provide results in a timely enough fashion. Commonly, emergency room and obstetrical personnel would be unable to test a patient before providing necessary care. Kelen (Kelen et al. 1988a) found that 13% of the patients entering the Johns Hopkins Emergency Room with penetrating trauma were seropositive and that unprotected exposure to body fluids occurred in 84% of the cases (Kelen et al. 1988b).

The use of the "Universal Precautions" (Table 1-5), where caution is used when handling the blood and body fluids from all patients, should minimize the risk of exposure to all blood-borne pathogens. Sharp objects of all kinds must be handled with extreme caution, since these items clearly pose the greatest risk to the worker. Adverse exposures to the blood and body fluids from any patient should be treated immediately following an established policy that includes employee first aid, serological medical screening with proper follow-up, and evaluation of the exposure source (Centers for Disease Control 1987d). The use of antiretroviral drugs for treatment of adverse exposure is currently under study and may ultimately prove effective.

Table 1-5 Universal Precautions Summary

Use caution with blood and body fluids from **all** patients.
Gloves should be used when there is a high likelihood of blood and body fluids contacting hands.
Gowns should be used when there is a high likelihood of blood and body fluids contacting exposed skin.
Masks and eyewear should be used when there is a high likelihood of blood and body fluids splashing onto the face.
All sharp items should be handled carefully—do not bend, cut, or recap needles.
Give first aid, contact the supervisor, and contact employee health for all adverse exposures to blood or body fluids from any patient.
Clean all blood spills with an approved disinfectant.
Follow hospital policy for waste and linen disposal.
Train all employes on Universal Precautions who are performing tasks that have potential for exposure to blood and body fluids as they begin to work.
Monitor compliance and retrain those workers who are noncompliant.
Provide adequate supplies of barriers for employees.
Establish an employee health program that provides access to appropriate monitoring and counseling.

The CDC recognized the importance of involving employers in the implementation of their "Universal Precautions" guidelines and recommended that employers take responsibility for ensuring compliance from their workers. The CDC also recommended that employers train new employees, as well as current workers, about the epidemiology, transmission, and prevention of HIV and HBV infections, and about the proper use of barriers. Employers are also responsible for providing necessary barriers and equipment to allow employees to follow the "Universal Precautions" adequately. When employers identify noncompliant workers, they must have an established plan for retraining and disciplining them (Centers for Disease Control 1987d).

Shortly after the CDC published their guidelines for "Universal Precautions," the Occupational Safety and Health Administration (OSHA) of the Department of Labor (DOL) published an advisory notice entitled "Protection against Occupational Exposure to Hepatitis B Virus and Human Immunodeficiency Virus" in the *Federal Register*. The DOL called for healthcare employers to provide appropriate safeguards for their employees. According to the OSHA/

DOL notice, employers are legally responsible for providing training and appropriate equipment for their workers. Health care worker tasks associated with a likelihood of exposure to blood or body fluids are to be categorized I, II, or III (decreasing levels of risk for exposure). Standard operating procedures must be developed that include identification of necessary barriers and/or equipment. Engineering controls are to be developed whenever possible to minimize unnecessary exposure to blood and body fluids. Employee medical care including access to voluntary HBV vaccination, serological monitoring as requested by the worker for HBV and HIV following parenteral exposure, and proper care and counseling following adverse exposures are required.

OSHA began a program of enforcement shortly after the *Federal Register* publication on the "Universal Precautions." Their program includes a system for responding to employee complaints regarding employer noncompliance with these guidelines. OSHA has also initiated a program of spot checks to assure worker protection.

Conclusions

Evidence now exists that the risk for occupationally acquired HIV infection for healthcare workers is low. No matter how small, however, this risk deserves respect from all workers. The healthcare profession has always contended with occupational risks. The need to change old behaviors that place workers at risk may prove to be the most difficult task facing healthcare workers in the coming years. Fear and anxiety must be minimized by educating and providing protection to workers.

References

Barré-Sinoussi F., et al. 1983. Isolation of a T-lymphotropic retrovirus from a patient at risk for the acquired immunodeficiency syndrome. *Science* 220: 868–871.

Castro K.G., et al. 1988. Investigations of AIDS patients with no previously identified risk factors. *Journal of the American Medical Association* 259: 1338–1342.

Centers for Disease Control. 1981. *Pneumocystis* pneumonia. *Morbidity and Mortality Weekly Report* 30: 250–252.

Centers for Disease Control. 1984. Hepatitis B Vaccine: Evidence confirming lack of AIDS transmission. *Morbidity and Mortality Weekly Report* 33: 685–686.

Centers for Disease Control. 1985a. Provisional Public Health Service interagency recommendations for screening donated blood and plasma for antibody to the virus causing acquired immunodeficiency syndrome. *Morbidity and Mortality Weekly Report* 34: 1–5.

Centers for Disease Control. 1985b. Recommendations for preventing transmission of infection with human T-lymphotropic virus type III/lymphadenopathy associated virus in the workplace. *Morbidity and Mortality Weekly Report* 34: 681–695.

Centers for Disease Control. 1986a. Acquired immunodeficiency syndrome (AIDS) in western Palm Beach County, Florida. *Morbidity and Mortality Weekly Report* 35: 609–613.

Centers for Disease Control. 1986b. Apparent transmission of human T-lymphotropic virus type III/lymphadenopathy-associated virus from a child to a mother providing healthcare. *Morbidity and Mortality Weekly Report* 35: 76–79.

Centers for Disease Control. 1986c. Safety of therapeutic immune globulin preparations with respect to transmission of human T-lymphotropic virus type III/lymphadenopathy-associated virus infection. *Morbidity and Mortality Weekly Report* 35: 231–233.

Centers for Disease Control. 1987a. Human immunodeficiency virus infection in the United States. *Morbidity and Mortality Weekly Report* 36: 801–804.

Centers for Disease Control. 1987b. Public Health Service guidelines for counseling and antibody testing to prevent HIV infection and AIDS. *Morbidity and Mortality Weekly Report* 36: 509–515.

Centers for Disease Control. 1987d. Recommendations for prevention of HIV transmission in healthcare settings. *Morbidity and Mortality Weekly Report* 36 (Supplement): 1S–18S.

Centers for Disease Control. 1987e. Update: Human immunodeficiency virus infections in healthcare workers exposed to blood of infected patients. *Morbidity and Mortality Weekly Report* 36: 285–289.

Centers for Disease Control. 1988a. 1988 Agent summary statement for human immunodeficiency virus and report on laboratory–acquired infection with human immunodeficiency virus. *Morbidity and Mortality Weekly Report* 37 (Supplement): S–4.

Centers for Disease Control. 1988b. *AIDS Weekly Surveillance Report* December 5.

Centers for Disease Control. 1988c. Update: Acquired immunodeficiency syndrome and human immunodeficiency virus infection among healthcare workers. *Morbidity and Mortality Weekly Report* 37: 229–239.

Centers for Disease Control. 1988d. Update: Universal precautions for prevention of transmission of human immunodeficiency virus, hepatitis B virus, and other blood-borne pathogens in healthcare settings. *Morbidity and Mortality Weekly Report* 37: 377–388.

Curran, J.W., et al. 1988. Epidemiology of HIV infection and AIDS in the United States. *Science* 239: 610–616.

Department of Labor, Department of Health and Human Services. 1987. HBV/HIV. *Federal Register* 52: 41818–41824. Washington, D.C.: Government Printing Offices.

Elmslie, K., and J.V. O'Shaughnessy. 1987. National surveillance program on occupational exposure to HIV among health-care workers in Canada. *Canadian Disease Weekly Report* 13: 163–166.

Fauci, A.S. 1988. The human immunodeficiency virus: Infectivity and mechanisms of pathogenesis. *Science* 239: 617–622.

Fischl, M.A., et al. 1987. Evolution of heterosexual partners, children, and household contacts of adults with AIDS. *Journal of the American Medical Association.* 257: 640–644.

Friedland, G.H., and R.S. Klein. 1987. Transmission of the human immunodeficiency virus. *New England Journal of Medicine* 317: 1125–1135.

Friedland, G.H., et al. 1987. Additional evidence for lack of transmission of HIV infection to household contacts of AIDS patients. Abstract TP.67. Presented at the 3rd International Conference on AIDS, June, Washington, D.C.

Gallo, R.C., et al. 1984. Frequent detection of cytopathic retrovirus (HTLV-III) from patients with AIDS and at risk for AIDS. *Science* 224: 500–503.

Gerberding, J.L., and D.K. Henderson. 1987. Design of rational infection control policies for human immunodeficiency virus infection. *Journal of Infectious Diseases* 156: 861–864.

Gerberding, J.L. et al. 1987. Risk of transmitting the human immunodeficiency virus, cytomegalovirus, and hepatitis B virus to healthcare workers exposed to patients with AIDS and AIDS-related conditions. *Journal of Infectious Diseases* 156: 1–8.

Gioananni, P., et al. 1988. HIV infection acquired by a nurse. *European Journal of Epidemiology* 4: 119–120.

Glatt, A.E., K. Chirgivia, and S.H. Landesman. 1988. Treatment of infections associated with human immunodeficiency virus. *New England Journal of Medicine* 318: 1439–1448.

Goedert, J.J., et al. 1986. Three year incidence of AIDS in five cohorts of HTLV-III-infected risk group members. *Science* 231: 992–995.

Grint, P., and M. McEvoy. 1985. Two associated cases of the acquired immune deficiency syndrome (AIDS). PHLS *Communicable Disease Report* 85142: 42–44.

Handsfield, H.H., M.J. Cummings, and P.D. Swenson. 1987. Prevalence of antibody to human immunodeficiency virus and hepatitis B surface antigen in blood samples submitted to a hospital laboratory. *Journal of the American Medical Association* 258: 3395–3397.

Henderson, D.K., B.J. Fahey, and M.E. Willy. 1988. Frequency and intensity of cutaneous exposures to blood and body fluids among healthcare providers in a referral hospital. Abstract 9017. Presented at the 4th International Conference on AIDS, Stockholm, Sweden, June.

Henderson, D.K., et al. 1988. Longitudinal assessment of the risk for occupational/nosocomial transmission of human immunodeficiency virus, type I in healthcare workers (abstract). Presented at the 28th Interscience Conference on Antimicrobial Agents and Chemotherapy, Los Angeles, Oct.

Hernandez, E., et al. 1988. Risk of transmitting the HIV to healthcare workers (HCW) exposed to HIV infected body fluids. Abstract 9003. Presented at the 4th International Conference on AIDS, Stockholm, Sweden, June.

Hessol, N.A., et al. 1987. The natural history of human immunodeficiency virus infection in a cohort of homosexual and bisexual men. Abstract M.3.1. Presented at the 3rd International Conference on AIDS, Washington, D.C., June.

Kelen, G.D., et al. 1988a. Unrecognized human immunodeficiency virus infection in emergency department patients. *New England Journal of Medicine* 318: 1645–1650.

Kelen, G.D., et al. 1988b. Unrecognized HIV infection in general emergency patients. Abstract 9019. Presented at the 4th International Conference on Aids, June, Stockholm, Sweden.

Klein, R.S., et al. 1988. Low occupational risk of human immunodeficiency virus infection among dental professionals. *New England Journal of Medicine* 318: 86–90.

Kuhls, T.L., et al. 1987. Occupational risk of HIV, HBV, and HSV-2 infections in healthcare personnel caring for AIDS patients. *American Journal of Public Health* 77: 1306–1309.

Lifson, A.R. 1988. Do alternate modes for transmission of human immunodeficiency virus exist? *Journal of the American Medical Association* 259: 1353–1356.

Marcus, R. 1988. The Cooperative Needlestick Surveillance Group. CDC's healthcare workers surveillance project: An update. Abstract 9015. Presented at the 4th International Conference on AIDS, Stockholm, Sweden, June.

Marx, J.L. 1988. Multiplying genes by leaps and bounds. *Science* 240: 1408–1410.

McCray, E. 1986. The Cooperative Needlestick Surveillance Group. Occupational risk of the acquired immunodeficiency syndrome among healthcare workers. *New England Journal of Medicine* 314: 1127–1132.

McEvoy, M., et al. 1987. Prospective study of clinical, laboratory, and ancillary staff with accidental exposures to blood or body fluids from patients infected with HIV. *British Journal of Medicine* 294: 1595–1597.

Michelet, C., et al. 1988. Needlestick HIV infection in a nurse. Abstract 9010. Presented at the 4th International Conference on AIDS, Stockholm, Sweden, June.

1984. Needlestick transmission of HTLV-III from a patient infected in Africa. *Lancet* 2: 1376–1377.

Neisson-Vernant, C., et al. 1986. Needlestick HIV seroconversion in a nurse (letter). *Lancet* 2: 814.

Oskenhendler, E., et al. 1986. HIV infection with seroconversion after a superficial needlestick injury to the finger (letter). *New England Journal of Medicine* 315: 582.

Pizzocolo, G., et al. 1988. Risk of HIV and HBV infection after accidental needlestick. Abstract 9012. Presented at the 4th International Conference on AIDS, Stockholm, Sweden, June.

Ponce deLeon, R.S., G. Sanchez-Mejorada, and M. Zaidi-Jacobsen. 1988. AIDS in a blood bank technician. *Infection Control and Hospital Epidemiology* 9: 101–102.

Ramsey, K.M., E.N. Smith, and J.A. Reinarz. 1988. Prospective evaluation of 44 healthcare workers exposed to human immunodeficiency virus-1, with one seroconversion (abstract). *Clinical Research* 36: 22A.

Ranki, A., et al. 1987. Long latency precedes overt seroconversion in sexually transmitted human immunodeficiency virus infection. *Lancet* 2: 589–593.

Redfield, R.R., et al. 1985. Frequent transmission of HTLV-III among spouses of patients with AIDS-related complex and AIDS. *Journal of the American Medical Association* 253: 1571–1573.

Robinson, W.B. 1985. Hepatitis B virus and the delta agent. In *Principles and Practice of Infectious Diseases*. 2d. ed., ed. G.L. Mandell, R.G. Douglas, and J.E. Bennett, 1002–1029. New York: John Wiley & Sons, Inc.

Stricof, R.L., and D.L. Morse. 1986. HTLV-III/LAV seroconversion following a deep intramuscular needlestick injury (letter). *New England Journal of Medicine* 314: 1115.

U.S. Public Health Service. 1986. Coolfont Report: A Public Health Service plan for prevention of AIDS and the AIDS virus. *Public Health Reports* 101: 341–348. Washington, D.C.: Government Printing Office.

Ward, J.W., et al. 1988. Transmission of human immunodeficiency virus by blood transfusion screened as negative for HIV antibody. *New England Journal of Medicine* 318: 473–478.

Weiss, S.H., et al. 1985. HTLV-III infection among healthcare workers. Association with needle-stick injuries. *Journal of the American Medical Association* 254: 2089–2093.

Weiss, S.H., et al. 1988. Risk of human immunodeficiency virus (HIV-1) infection among laboratory workers. *Science* 239: 68–71.

Wormser, G.P., et al. 1988. Human immunodeficiency virus infections: Considerations for healthcare workers. *Bulletin of the New York Academy of Medicine* 64: 203–215.

CHAPTER 2

A Personal AIDS Story

G. M. "Missy" LeClaire

In the beginning there was pure confusion about my husband, Jim. What could be wrong? Why is he so sick? What about the weight loss, the night sweats, the fatigue, the personality changes? How about the awful infection in his mouth? How long will it take for him to recover? Will he be out of work long? At least we have health insurance. Surely we are covered for any possible health crisis.

Then the diagnosis came—human T-cell lymphotropic (leukemia) virus type III (now included in the general terminology of human immunodeficiency virus (HIV-1)). So what does that mean? Hodgkin's disease? Leukemia? AIDS? AIDS!! What is AIDS? He isn't gay. He isn't an intravenous drug user. He is a merchant marine and has traveled around the world. He has even been to Africa. And, yes, he was in an automobile accident and received blood transfusions to save his life, but AIDS? This doesn't happen to regular people. We've only been married for six months. What happens now?

These were only some of the thoughts and questions that went through my mind as a family member of someone diagnosed with acquired immunodeficiency syndrome. The turmoil is never ending.

In April of 1986, after months of illness, Jim had required unrelated emergency surgery to repair urethral damage caused by an automobile accident he had been in. While he was a patient in a small community hospital, the care he received seemed inappropriate, to say the least. Among other things, food trays were left outside his room, his bed was never changed by hospital staff, he was rarely (if ever) touched by hospital staff (with or without gloves), and he was never washed by the staff. All of this was before he was finally diagnosed as having AIDS in late June.

After his release from this hospital, we ended up in the emergency room time after time for one problem after another. For one of these crises, I arranged to take him to a teaching hospital that had an AIDS unit. We made the four-hour trip with him lying in the back seat of the car with a catheter filled with blood. When we arrived at the teaching hospital, I felt as if we were in heaven. Here were people who understood and who were not afraid of Jim or of his illness.

The trauma we had been through had taken its toll on Jim. He had developed an extreme distrust of medical professionals. He could not understand why he had been treated so poorly at the first hospital and now at the new hospital, he couldn't understand why he was constantly being asked if he had ever had a homosexual experience or used intravenous drugs. He just wanted to get well and go home.

Jim's denial process was so strong that he had to be told the diagnosis twice within two weeks. He then spent four days with the bedcovers pulled up and over his head. He was 26 years old, newly wed, and had exciting career possibilities. He had a wonderful life ahead of him—or so he thought. He felt stigmatized by a disease so often associated with gay men and drug addicts. The thoughts that he would never have a child of his own, be captain of his own merchant sailing vessel, or even purchase a home were devastating and demoralizing. When you add to all of that the fear that he may have infected his wife along with all the anxieties and prejudices that surrounded his elementary knowledge of AIDS, you have an emotionally and physically dysfunctional human being.

Jim never suffered the typical opportunistic infections associated with AIDS. When he was released from his first AIDS-related hospitalization, we moved to the Washington, D.C. metropolitan area to be closer to proper medical and community support. Jim did well, initially. He gained weight, added color, tackled the candida with diet and medications, and was also able to control his depression with medications. This slight relief lasted from July until October of 1986.

The second week of October ended the respite. Jim turned from being a moody and sometimes agitated man into a volatile monster. He was sullen, angry, violent, frightened, and despondent all at one time, and then within a few minutes he would be laughing and loving. He was like Dr. Jekyll and Mr. Hyde. He would refuse to take his medications and instead drink alcohol or write "goodbye" notes. It was like living deep within the twilight zone with a husband I no longer knew.

After constant calls to his physicians and psychiatrists, I finally arranged for him to visit an outpatient clinic. When he was approached about entering the hospital for psychological and neurological tests, he ran away from the hospital. He was found later in the parking lot of this large inner-city hospital. He told the doctors that he was going to go live in the woods. There he knew he would be happy and could die peacefully.

A four-week stay in two different psychiatric institutions followed this altercation. The first accepted him with complete knowledge of his AIDS diagnosis. However, I soon realized that the staff and administration had little or no knowledge of AIDS or AIDS dementia complex. I was called on a daily basis to answer such questions as how I laundered his clothing or washed his dishes. Jim's primary psychiatrist also asked me what they should do if he became violent.

After a few days of this kind of communication, I began to search for a hospital that would accommodate him in a more humane and appropriate manner. I did find one that handled Jim and AIDS much more professionally. Again, there was still very little up-to-date knowledge of the neurological ravages of AIDS. I was told by the doctor that Jim was depressed because he had AIDS and that his irrational behavior was caused by authority problems stemming from childhood disagreements with his mother. Furthermore, I was told that he needed two or three years of intense psychotherapy to overcome all of this—a recommendation given to a man whose life expectancy was less than a year. However, with the help of therapy, group support, and antidepressants Jim was eventually able to make some strides in his outlook and seemed intent on having quality time with me.

After many discussions with the staff at the hospital, I decided to take Jim home. Treatment would continue on an outpatient basis with a Washington psychiatrist whose speciality was the various psychological and neurological disorders associated with AIDS. I could not foresee significant improvements, and our insurance funds were being depleted. I also felt that Jim should be allowed to enjoy whatever time he had left at home. While he was in the hospital he had gained back 30 pounds and was very close to his normal weight.

He came home to a warm reception by me and my parents shortly after Thanksgiving. All was well. He seemed to be able to keep his "quality" resolutions and was well enough to make a trip to upstate New York to visit his family where he healed old wounds with his mother and was received with love by all. We even took a side trip to Montreal—a kind of a second honeymoon. It was a marvelous vacation. He tired easily but was cheery and seemed reasonably healthy.

Two weeks later, on Christmas day, Jim awoke at home to open gifts with our family, but he was so fatigued that he went to bed right after breakfast and never made it to Christmas dinner. He was rarely out of bed after Christmas, and the only time he left the house was for visits to the psychiatrist's office. By the end of January, he was despondent and had no short-term memory at all. Whether this was due to medications or to physical/neurological problems was not certain, but I knew he was failing. His doctor suggested a hospital stay, and this time Jim was more than willing to go.

The seven days in the hospital were a nightmare. Jim was a terrible patient. He was agitated and aggravated by everything and everyone. The nurses had a hard time understanding this seemingly healthy looking young man who was being so difficult. He would ask questions over and over. He would forget that he had received medications and ask for them again. He wold forget that he had eaten and wonder if he was ever going to be fed. He had a new primary physician, and neither knew the other. This doctor was an excellent physician, well versed in the complex health issues of AIDS, however, his personality was a bit gruff and abrupt.

Finally, the test results were in. I was told (in Jim's presence) to line up a hospice service. When I asked why, the doctor replied coldly, "because he's got less than six months."

Jim was diagnosed with dementia. How long had I suspected? Would an earlier dementia diagnosis have made a difference? Jim was also diagnosed with *Mycobacterium avium-intracellulare* (MAI), a tuberculean type of infection that enters the bone marrow and ravages the body. The only treatments available for it are experimental and painful.

As we left the hospital, Jim asked that he never have to return. "I'd like to die at home, if you can handle it," he said. I promised to keep him with me at home if I could manage, regardless of the personal or monetary cost. As the weeks wore on, I regretted my decision many times.

This was extremely difficult work. At first, Jim was capable of getting up and around. He could walk to the bathroom, feed himself, and look after his own personal care. He also finally seemed at peace with himself and the world. He was a loving husband, a thankful man, and happy to be with someone who loved and cared for him—what a delightful change!

Physically, however, he became progressively worse. In a matter of weeks he was totally bedridden and required 24-hour care. He grew more and more demented, was not able to eat, and lost nearly 100 pounds. Due to the dementia and the narcotics he was given for pain control, Jimmy was "in another world" most of the time—fortunately. The MAI infection caused him to have extended fevers from 104° to 106°. I thought a person would die immediately when his temperature went that high. Chills preceded fevers that seemed to raise his body from the bed and were followed by sweats that would soak through the sheets. This would happen between five and seven time a day—every day.

My main sources of help and support were my mother and father; they kept food on the table, the sheets washed, and my spirits up. I had contracted the services of a local hospice to care for Jim on an at-home basis. However, as it turned out, the hospice staff was more of a support system for me than for Jim. There was very little anyone could do for him beyond what I was doing already, except control his pain. I was taught to give him pain injections every two hours around the clock. Prior training had taught me how to change our bed with him in it, how to protect against bedsores, how to rub him down with alcohol to reduce fevers, and how to give him a bed bath. I found the strength and know-how to fight all the other battles and crises in the love of my husband, faith in God, and faith in myself.

On April 19, 1987 Jim slipped into unconsciousness. He died at home in my arms on April 22, over a year after he first became ill. I was glad it was over—for both of us.

CHAPTER 3

Psychosocial Issues

John Maddix

AIDS has become the disease of the 1980s. As of December, 1988, approximately 80,996 persons have been diagnosed with AIDS (Centers for Disease Control 1988). Of that number, over half have died. The Centers for Disease Control (CDC) also report that one to two million Americans have already been infected with the human immunodeficiency virus (HIV) and that this number could jump to at least 5 million within 5 to 10 years.

The effects of AIDS have been devastating on the gay community in this country. For tens of thousands of gay men, the death of loved ones and friends has become a regular occurrence. For most of these men, the stress of constant grief is amplified by fear that the next cough or skin blemish will signal the beginning of their own battle with AIDS.

This chapter examines how the AIDS epidemic affects gay men, primarily those with HIV disease, and it will look at how society, family, and friends affect this population. Although AIDS has affected various other groups, the focus will be on gay men because most of the psychosocial research to date has studied this population and because gay men represent the large majority of people with HIV disease. In the last two years a significant amount of literature has been devoted to the psychosocial needs of persons with AIDS, and there is an increasing number of studies focusing on the psychosocial needs of HIV-positive persons. Other data have been extrapolated from studies done with cancer patients and related to people with HIV disease. This chapter will look at some ethical crises faced by people with HIV disease and some policy questions.

31

The complexity of problems confronting people with AIDS and the psychological terror it engenders set this disease apart from virtually every other contemporary public health problem. Its onset affects every aspect of a person's life. It creates serious problems for those with whom the patient has personal, intimate, familial, or occupational ties. It produces difficult patient management issues for provider institutions and community agencies, and it raises basic ethical issues of how society views and treats people with AIDS-related conditions. It illustrates the problems of how governmental agencies respond to and pay for catastrophic illness in this society, and it arouses issues of AIDS panic in a society that believes the disease is more contagious than it actually is.

There is no known cure for AIDS even though there seems to be a handful of people who are alive and well after five years. Currently, there are treatments for specific conditions, and the discovery of azidothymidine (AZT) has raised the hopes of thousands of persons with AIDS-related conditions. However, these persons are still confronted with the fact that as yet there are no treatments for the immunodeficiency itself. The disease and its sequelae are overwhelming and physically debilitating. The transition from being a young, active, vigorous person to a weakened, symptom-racked, possibly dying person, often over the course of only a few weeks or months, is devastating even to contemplate.

AIDS is a severely stigmatizing lethal disease that puts at risk the health and survival of individuals in already highly stigmatized populations (Kowalewski 1985). Antibody-positive persons suffer a blow to not only their physical being, but also to their self-image, and often they present symptoms of severe anxiety and depression (Morin, Charles, and Malyon 1984). The knowledge that they are antibody-positive causes many persons to enter into a state of crisis.

According to Hans Selye (1975), stress is the nonspecific response of the body to any demand made upon it. Stress requires adaptation to a problem, irrespective of what that problem may be. Everything to which a human being is exposed produces a nonspecific increase in the need to perform adaptive functions and thereby to reestablish normalcy. This is independent of the specific activity that caused the rise in requirements. The nonspecific demand for activity as such is the essence of stress. From the point of view of its stress-producing or stressor activity, it is immaterial whether the agency or situation faced is pleasant or unpleasant; all that counts is the intensity of the demand for readjustment or adaptation. Selye emphasizes that stress is a normal event. In fact, he states that life without stress equals death.

Selye states that every disease causes a certain amount of stress since it imposes demands for adaptation upon the organism. In turn, stress plays some role in the development of every disease; it effects, for better or worse, add to the specific changes characteristic of the disease in question. It is important to note that all people react to stress differently and use different coping mechanisms to deal with it. What is stressful to some may not be stressful to others. Selye states that prevention should not try to avoid stress, but should recognize individual typical responses to it and moderate behavior accordingly.

In an article in the *Washington Post* (April 9, 1986), Sally Squires described studies indicating that the relationship between stress and disease is not a simple cause-and-effect connection but rather a complex equation that can change with the situation and individual. High levels of stress may promote illness by altering the immune system and placing an added load on the heart and blood vessels. The article also presented several studies relating stress to decreased immune functioning. The implications for gay men exposed to the AIDS antibody are enormous. If stress can decrease immune functioning in persons with intact immune systems, then a person with an already existing immunosuppressing virus may be more susceptible to AIDS and other illnesses.

There is a growing body of cancer-related literature which suggests that the psychological reactions of persons with cancer influence their physical well-being and ultimate prognosis. Persons with cancer frequently find that their own anxiety is escalated by the negative attitudes of others, thus placing a burden on them in addition to that imposed by the disease itself (Verwoerdt 1966; Wortman 1983). Some patients experience overwhelming feelings of powerlessness, loss of control, and inability to cope (Bean et al. 1980). Because of the fears that cancer generates, patients often experience the course of their illness in relative isolation (Bilick and Nuland 1981). In Young's very comprehensive article devoted to support groups and cancer, she cites studies by Bilick and Nuland that report a composite model of the mind-body unity concept discussed by

LeShan (1977) and by Simonton and Matthews-Simonton (1981) and states: "When cancer develops it is not as a result of the cancer cell's inherent power, but because of a breakdown in the immune system" (1986, 4). In this approach, cancer is conceptualized to be weak, and the deficit is in the immune system's normal functioning.

In an article by Reuben (1986), Louse Hay, who maintained that she directed her own healing and rid herself of vaginal cancer, states that the positive or negative attitudes of people with cancer or with any life-threatening disease have an affect on the immune system which is considered critical in the fight to live. This evidence supports the theory that HIV-positive persons can do something to improve their immune functioning by reducing stress and increasing positivity in their lives.

The amount of stress in the life of a gay man affected by the disease can be enormously high. Holland and Tross (1985) identify five psychological symptoms common to people with AIDS: anxiety, depression, sense of isolation, reduced support, and anger. The major form of psychological distress is a preoccupation with illness with the potential for a rapidly declining course to death. The same existential issues raised by a diagnosis of cancer and other diseases with high fatal outcome are raised by a diagnosis of AIDS (Morin et al. 1984; Weisman and Worden 1976). An infected person's mood may be characterized by sadness, hopelessness, and helplessness. Guilt, low self-esteem, worthlessness, and anticipatory grief are common with social withdrawal and isolation. Guilt may further magnify the sense of isolation and estrangement many gay men have experienced throughout much of their lives (Cassens 1985).

Antibody-positive persons are in a unique position in that they may suffer severe consequences if they reveal their antibody status. The losses of jobs, friends, family, health insurance, etc. are very real consequences. As antibody-positive status is associated with homosexuality, such revelations involve issues of society's homophobia, and infected persons are often denied the comfort, sympathy, and empathy offered to persons with other potentially fatal conditions just when they may be most vulnerable (Cassens 1985).

Perhaps the most horrifying recent discovery is that the mean latency time from exposure to AIDS to diagnosis may be considerably longer than previously thought. In a study of transfusion-associated people with AIDS, Curran et al. (1984) determined that the observed mean is 26.6 months from the initial infection to the virus to the development of full-blown case of AIDS. Lawrence et al. (1985) calculated an estimated mean latency time of nearly five to seven years. For those infected with the virus the meaning is clear: there is no end to the daily worry of if and when one may come down with AIDS. Current studies show that the latency period may extend to 10 years or more. In a hepatitis B vaccine study conducted on gay men in San Francisco, over 77% of those who are HIV-positive have developed symptoms, most of whom have not yet developed a full-blown case of AIDS (Storrs 1987). What is clear is that the longer a person is antibody-positive, the more likely it is that he or she will develop symptoms and full-blown AIDS.

Ethical Issues

The many and varied ethical issues related to AIDS and people with AIDS-related conditions are complicated, emotionally charged, and often without precedent. The needs of people exposed to HIV are, or perhaps appear to be, in conflict with larger societal issues. Do issues of confidentiality outweigh the right of people in society to know whether a person is antibody-positive? For example, do co-workers, especially healthcare workers and teachers, for example, need to be informed of a person's antibody status? Do physicians have the right to conduct HIV tests on people whom they suspect or know are in high risk groups without their consent? In counseling large numbers of people who have tested positive for the HIV antibody, helping persons are continually confronted with questions of whether such clients should continue to have sex, and, if so, whether they should tell their prospective partners about their antibody status. Does the state have the right and obligation to track down partners of persons with AIDS-related conditions? The list of ethical dilemmas continues to grow and expand.

For gay men, the issues are complicated even more by the fact that homosexual activity between consenting adults is a felony in many jurisdictions. In fact, the United States Supreme Court (Bowers v. Hardwick 1986) recently upheld a Georgia law that allows states to regulate the private sexual activity of its citizens and to distinguish between "normal" heterosexual activities and "abnormal" homosexual activities. The Court ruled that homosexual sodomy could not be protected by the right of privacy in the Constitution. The criminalization of gay men and women, especially gay men with AIDS, leads to increased stress levels and only exacerbates their fear.

Confidentiality of a person's HIV antibody status is particularly important because of the potential personal, social, and economic harms that may result from disclosure of this information. Thus, blood banks, healthcare personnel, and researchers have sought to ensure the confidentiality of records. Federal regulations exist to protect the confidentiality of drug and alcohol records (Federal Register 1975). Federal regulations also exist to protect the identity of research subjects (Federal Register 1979). There are no equivalent federal protections for doctor-patient communications. There is a common-law doctor-patient privilege that protects the confidentiality of records even against the judicial process unless overridden by a compelling state interest. In the case of AIDS, is there such a compelling interest?

In order to understand further the process of decision making from an ethical model, the issue of HIV-positive persons' responsibility to inform or not to inform potential sexual partners will be explored here according to the principles of utilitarian and deontological theory. Beauchamp and Childress (1983) state that utilitarianism refers to the moral theory that there is one and only one basic principle in ethics—the principle of utility. This principle asserts that in all circumstances, persons ought to produce the greatest possible balance of value over disvalue for all persons affected (or the least possible balance of disvalue if only bad results can be brought about). Utilitarianism looks at morality in terms of the consequences, or, stated in another way, all acts should promote the greatest good for the greatest number. By contrast, deontological theories, according to Beauchamp and Childress (1983), hold that some features of acts other than, or in addition to, their consequences make them right or wrong.

People with HIV disease must make decisions based on these principles. Does the fact that an HIV-positive person has "very safe sex" with a person based on the belief that his or her partner will not be at risk of contagion (utilitarian) outweigh the principle that high risk persons need to be honest about their actions (deontological)? That is, does the principle of honesty outweigh the risk of possible outright rejection in those acts with minimal or no risk involved? When does one tell a partner that he or she is HIV-positive? Would one only tell after the partner has made a commitment of some kind to the person with an HIV infection? The utilitarian might say that the very possibility of contagion should preclude any form of sexual contact, whereas the deontologist might say that the fact that the person has taken precautions to avoid the possibility of contagion might justify some sexual acts, e.g., there is no justification for a person to indulge in sexual acts which offer no protection to the other person. The ethical dilemma lies of course in that gray area in which there is an element of risk.

Beauchamp and Childress (1983, 59) state that "the most general idea of personal autonomy is still that of self-governance, being one's own person with constraints either by another's action or by psychological or physical limitations." The autonomous person determines his or her course of action in accordance with a plan chosen by himself or herself. The questions faced by HIV-positive persons are whether they are causing harm by even having safer sex with a person, and whether they should base their actions on this principle.

The principle of nonmaleficence refers to the noninfliction of harm and the removal of harmful conditions, while beneficence, according to Beauchamp and Childress (1983, 107-179), is far reaching because it requires positive steps to help others. It is often difficult to distinguish between the two. William Frankena (1963) held that the principle of beneficence includes four elements: one ought not to inflict evil or harm; one ought to prevent evil or harm; one ought to remove evil; and one ought to do or promote good. To what extent does one's refusal to discuss one's antibody status infringe on the right of the other person to make decisions about his or her life?

The ultimate fears that an antibody-positive person faces are the possibility of infecting another person and the guilt and uncertainty this may cause as well as possible rejection by potential partners. In informing potential partners, the antibody-positive person also runs the risk that this person may not respect his or her confidentiality. If one practices safer sex techniques with the understanding that these present minimal or no risk to potential partners, does one have the obligation to inform them? What is an accepted risk?

The above dilemma illustrates how deontological and utilitarian theoretical frameworks can be used to make ethical decisions and can be applied to any number of ethical questions posed by AIDS in this society. The above discussion only touches on the complexity of one major issue people with AIDS-related conditions may bring to a support group or to helping persons. Being confronted with such decisions may cause the HIV-infected person incredible stress and conflict, especially in a society in which some would like to deny them the right to make these decisions.

Lack of Policy

The major policy questions of AIDS center around the treatment of persons with AIDS-related conditions and the development of effective ways to curb the spread of the virus, and the funding of these activities. Central to an issue as large as AIDS is which private and/or public agencies are going to develop programs to carry out the above policies, and perhaps more importantly, who is going to fund such programs?

When the virus was perceived to affect mainly gay male and intravenous drug user communities, the public's response was to decry the immorality of those affected and to blame them for the disease. Little assistance was provided by nongay agencies at the beginning stages of the epidemic. As it has become clearer that AIDS is a virus that is not limited by sexual orientation or intravenous drug use but threatens all people, the federal, state, and local governments and private organizations have begun to debate how to provide services, and to whom.

Even the scientific-medical community was slow to respond to this epidemic. Edward Brandt, former assistant secretary for health stated that some members of the scientific community were questioning whether or not to study AIDS because it had become a gay rights issue (Talbot and Bush 1985). This point was backed up in the same article by several other notable researchers.

The hallmark of a health emergency like AIDS is its unpredictability. Therefore, initial research resources have to be re-budgeted.

In an earlier time, the issues before Congress and the President were whether they were going to fund programs for AIDS and if so to what level. Today, the debate centers on which health-related budgets have to be reduced in order to increase funding for AIDS research, education, and treatment (Harding 1987). The competition for federal dollars has begun, Peter is robbing Paul to pay the bills, and no one is happy.

The fear of many gay people and others is that as it becomes more evident that heterosexuals who are not intravenous drug users are not going to be affected in large numbers, the private and governmental sectors will be less willing to provide adequate funding to care for thousands of gay men and intravenous drug users. People with AIDS may face the loss of their income and insurance. The stressful issues then become whether the government will provide enough income for them to live; whether it will provide adequate and accessible healthcare; and whether it will pay for medications, including experimental drugs. Because more than 50% of all people with AIDS lose a significant portion of their income, these worries may create more stress in their lives.

Homophobia

Spokesmen for the gay community are greatly concerned that AIDS will renew the feelings of hostility, fear, and anger of the past within the heterosexual community as well as the gay community (Mayer and Pizer 1983). Gay men are worried that the reaction to AIDS will lead to a loss of personal freedom and that the open expression of the gay life-style will become unacceptable once again. This fear is an appropriate one since AIDS is an issue in legal cases involving gay men. In the state of Texas, a gay man charged with sexual assault and sodomy was required to submit to an HIV antibody test solely on the basis of his sexual orientation (Shelvin v. Patricia Lykos 1987). In addition, there are some gay and straight individuals who also perceive AIDS to be a punishment gay men are receiving for their "sinful" behavior, an attitude faced by other risk groups whose members feel considerable social stigma.

Gay men are less visible, however, than some of the other risk groups, and their lack of visibility is clearly self-maintained. Gay males may repress certain aspects of their life-style so they may incorporate themselves into the mainstream culture in response to the homophobic attitudes of the society. These factors all lead to an increase of stress that is environmentally induced. A recent Gallup poll showed that only 33% of the American public thought that homosexual acts should be decriminalized versus 44% in 1985—a drop of 11 percentage points that Jeff Levy, Chair of the National Gay Task Force (Harding 1986), attributes to AIDS hysteria.

Homophobia is defined as negative attitudes toward gay men and lesbians based on prejudice or on an experience that is colored by prejudice (Weinberg 1972). Internalized homophobia refers to the prejudicial attitudes held by the larger society about homosexuality that gay men and women have incorporated and internalized. In addition, gay men and lesbians, like racial minorities, frequently become the object of social oppression and as a result adopt characteristics that are judged to be "different" and "inferior" (Pillard 1982).

An increase in internalized homophobia is one of the clear presenting psychological reactions to the threat of AIDS for the gay man. AIDS occurs in risk groups that are already so oppressed by society that one can refer to them as satellite cultures (Hirsch and Enlow 1984). Such cultures develop in opposition to the mainstream, and individuals in these cultures can assimilate the negative reactions to their own characteristics. Within the gay community, the homophobic response to AIDS is amplified, incorporated into the perception of themselves, and internalized into the individuals' negative self-image.

An increasing number of studies have measured healthcare workers' knowledge and attitudes about people with AIDS. The *British Journal of Medicine* (Morton and McManus 1986) presented a study demonstrating that attitudes to AIDS and its treatment among a group of preclinical students did not correlate with knowledge about the condition but instead were related to attitudes in general concerning homosexuality. Morton and McManus (1986) conclude that to reduce prejudice about AIDS and increase public awareness of the problems of persons with AIDS, there should be increased emphasis on general education about homosexuality rather than on the specific and factual details of the disease. In a study conducted

in 1985, Douglas, Kalman, and Kalman found a great deal of homophobia among doctors and nurses. In an article entitled "Stigmatization of AIDS Patients by Physicians," a group of researchers (Kelly
et al. 1987) found that physicians' attitudes, as measured by their
reactions to a leukemic patient and an AIDS patient described in
identical vignettes, were harsher and more judgmental toward the
AIDS portrayal. The physicians' reactions indicated that they were
much less willing to interact even in routine conversation with
people with AIDS.

Because physicians and other healthcare persons are required to
provide services for people with AIDS, the ramifications become
great. Will they provide adequate care and respond to the needs of
people with AIDS? Will such negative attitudes increase the stress
and anxiety levels of persons with HIV disease? In fact, many people
with HIV disease are reluctant to seek medical care because of
possible repercussions and prejudice. Health care institutions must
address squarely the issue of homophobia if they are to provide
quality care to large numbers of gay people.

Loss and Grief

Ours is a "death-denying society" (Kubler-Ross 1969). Because
our society emphasizes competence, adequacy, strength, and ac-
complishment, the bereaved are often prevented by their family and
friends from expressing their true feelings. This tendency is compounded for survivors of persons who have died from AIDS since
very few people may even know that the survivor is experiencing a
loss. His family, co-workers, neighbors, and even most of his gay
friends may not be aware of it.

Loss sets in motion a train of feelings called grief. According to
Simos,

> In grief, what is normal goes contrary to what we usually
> think of as good adjustments, namely, a rational approach to
> problem solving, the ability to cope with one's problem, a
> sense of organization and orderliness, an optimistic outlook
> and the capacity to relate in a constructive way to other
> people (Simos 1979, 14).

Many people do not understand this. Under the guise of being helpful, they may give conflicting messages to persons who are grieving, e.g., you'll feel better, cheer up, get on with life, find a new boyfriend, and so on. These are not bad or cruel messages, but they do communicate to the bereaved or to people with HIV disease that others may not want to deal with this emotion and that there is some artificial time limit as to when the grieving process should stop.

People with HIV disease may begin a process of grieving shortly after learning that they are HIV-positive. Many of them may be already grieving the loss of other friends. Other gay men are unsure of how to grieve for a lover because they have little or no history of how to mourn such a loss. They may wonder how much sorrow is appropriate given that theirs was not a socially, legally, or religiously recognized marriage relationship. Many gay men appear to minimize or avoid their grief. "No permission is given oneself to honor their relationships," says Judy Pollatsek of the St. Francis Center in Washington, D.C. (1987). She attributes this lack of permission to internalized homophobia. Aside from these issues, gay men face problems similar to those of many men in American culture in their inability and/or discomfort with expressing feelings.

To add to the stresses experienced by the death of a loved one or a diagnosis of one's own disease, many persons find that they have isolated themselves from their friends and other support systems. Illness, particularly if it is severe, usually creates a sense of distance, difference, or isolation (Kubler-Ross 1969). The seriousness of AIDS coupled with its association with socially disapproved sexual behavior and capped by uncertain risks of contagion by those associated with persons with AIDS, often produce extreme isolation and ostracism. Because the public is at best ambivalent about the disease and those affected by it, persons whose lives are impacted by HIV disease tend to be denied some of the psychological benefits given to survivors of other less stigmatizing diseases (Christ and Wiener 1985). A very important role of the helping person, therefore, is to assist these people to maintain an existing network of friends and acquaintances or to develop one in what Bloom (1981) refers to as natural helping networks. In the gay community such a linkage would be to gay/lesbian organizations or self-help groups. In most larger cities, local gay health agencies provide a wide range of services which may include bereavement groups.

Many authors have emphasized the pivotal role of the family in helping ill or bereaved persons cope with and work through grief. Such support for gay people by their families should not be taken for granted. Many gay people are in the closet to their families and others or may have been abandoned by them. Many families may accept the gay family member but not the lover or gay friends, which then becomes a source of conflict and stress. It is not uncommon for some families to abandon their children even on their deathbeds. Of course, most families are there for their sons, but their presence or support should not be assumed. Often, there may also have been conflict between lovers of people with AIDS and the family of the deceased over living arrangements, care, visitation, and power of attorney. Issues around families of origin need to be discussed and assessed. Many gay people refer to their closest friends as family and use them for support. Loss of a friend or lover to AIDS may stir up old issues of family which need to be dealt with during an illness or afterwards during the grieving process.

Conclusions

The psychosocial picture of someone faced with HIV disease is not good. They may face the stigma of AIDS by the larger society and the rejection that it implies. They may lose family or friends, jobs, housing, and children. In addition to all of this, they have to face all of the issues anyone else with a life-threatening illness faces.

What is remarkable is that a larger gay community has been there to assist gay men and other persons affected by HIV disease and AIDS. Organizations have been created, primarily by gay and lesbian people, in most larger cities and in many smaller ones, to assist people with HIV disease. Support groups have been formed, housing has been found, financial resources have been tapped, etc. At present, many nongay persons are actively engaged in the fight against bigotry and are working to ensure that people with AIDS receive compassionate and fair treatment.

As these changes occur, many gay people with AIDS have formed their own self-help organizations, such as the National Association of People with AIDS, with Washington's local chapter named Lifelink. As people with AIDS become more empowered, they are forming self-help groups focusing on holistic and nontraditional treatments for HIV disease. Throughout the United States buying clubs are being formed to purchase medicines not available in this country. Groups of people with AIDS are testifying before Congress, state legislatures, and the AIDS Commission. Thousands of people with AIDS are involved in organizations seeking to educate the public about how to prevent this disease.

AIDS is going to be on this planet for decades to come. If this country is to meet the needs of growing numbers of people with AIDS and AIDS-related conditions and also people who love them, these issues need attention. The American people need not only to listen to the suffering of people with AIDS, they need to respond appropriately and with compassion and fairness.

References

Bean, G., et al. 1980. Coping mechanisms of cancer patients: A study of 33 patients receiving chemotherapy. *CA: Cancer Journal for Clinicians* 30: 256–259.

Beauchamp, T.L., and J.R. Childress. 1983. *Principles of biomedical ethics.* 2d ed. New York: Oxford University Press, Inc.

Bilick, H.A., and W. Nuland. 1981. A psychological model in the treatment of cancer patients. *In The psychotherapeutic treatment of cancer patients,* ed. J. G. Goldberg, 58–70. New York: Free Press.

Bloom, M. 1981. *Primary prevention: The possible science,* Englewood Cliffs, NJ: Prentice-Hall, Inc.

Cassens, B. 1985. Social consequences of the acquired immunodeficiency syndrome. *Annals of Internal Medicine* 103: 768–774.

Centers for Disease Control. 1988. AIDS Weekly Surveillance Report, December 19.

Christ, G., and L. Weiner. 1985. Psychosocial issues of AIDS. *In AIDS: Etiology, diagnosis, treatment and prevention,* ed. Devita, V.T., Hellman, S., and Rosenberg, S.A. 275–297. Philadelphia: J.B. Lippincott Co.

Curran, J.W., et al. 1984. Acquired immunodeficiency syndrome (AIDS) associated with transfusions. *New England Journal of Medicine* 310: 69–75.

Department of Health and Human Services. 1975. Confidentiality of alcohol and drug abuse patients records. *Federal Register* 40: 27802–27821. Washington, D.C.: Government Printing Office.

Department of Health and Human Services. 1979. Protection of identity of research subjects. *Federal Register* 44: 20382–20387. Washington, D.C., Government Printing Office.

Douglas, C., C. Kalman, and T. Kalman. 1985. Homophobia among physicians and nurses: An empirical study. *Hospital and Community Psychiatry* 36: 1309–1311.

Frankena, W. 1963. *Introduction to ethics.* Englewood Cliffs, NJ: Prentice-Hall, Inc.

Harding, R. 1986. Recent polls show drop in public support on gay issues. *The Washington Blade* 21 Nov., 3.

Harding, R. 1987. Kennedy, Weicker fight for adequate funding. *The Washington Blade* 16 Jan., 1.

Hirsch, D.A., and R. Enlow. 1984. The effects of the acquired immune deficiency syndrome on gay lifestyle and the gay individual. *Annals of the New York Academy of Sciences* 437: 272–282.

Holland, J.C., and S. Tross. 1985. The psychosocial and neuropsychiatric sequelae of the acquired immunodeficiency syndrome and related disorders. *Annals of Internal Medicine.* 103: 760–764.

Kelly, J., et al. 1987. Stigmatization of AIDS patients by physicians. *American Journal of Public Health.* 77: 789–791.

Kowalewski, M.R. 1985. Lepers in our midst: A stigmatized community deals with troubles from within. Unpublished manuscript.

Kubler-Ross, E. 1969. *On death and dying.* New York: Macmillan Publishing Company.

Lawrence, D., et al. 1985. A mode-based estimate of the average incubation and latency period for transfusion-associated AIDS. Paper presented at the International Conference on AIDS, Atlanta, GA. May, 1985.

LeShan, L. 1977. *You can fight for your life.* New York: M. Evans & Co. Inc.

Mayer, K., and J. Pizer. 1983. *The AIDS fact book,* 73–75. New York: Bantam Books.

Morin, S.F., K. Charles, and A. Malyon. 1984. The psychological impact of AIDS on gay men. *American Psychologist* 39: 1288–1293.

Morton, A.D., and I. McManus. 1986. Attitudes to and knowledge about the acquired immune deficiency syndrome: Lack of a correlation. *British Medical Journal* 293: 1212.

Pillard, R.D. 1982. Psychotherapeutic treatment for the invisible minority. *American Behavioral Scientist* (March/April): 25.

Pollatsek, J. 1987. Personal communication.

Reuben, C. 1986. AIDS: The promise of alternative treatments. *East-West* 16: 52–64.

Selye, H. 1975. *Stress without distress.* New York: The New American Library, Inc.

Simonton, O.C., and S. Matthews-Simonton. 1981. Cancer and stress: Counseling the cancer patient. *Medical Journal of Australia* 1: 679–683.

Simos, B. 1979. *A time to grieve: Loss as a universal human experience* 1–27, 244–251. New York: Family Service Association of America.

Squires, S. 1987. Learning to live with stress. 1986. *Washington Post* April 9.

Storrs, R. 1987. Insights on seropositivity. *The Documentation of AIDS Issues and Research Foundation, Inc.* Update 7 (Apr. 9): 1–2.

Talbot, D. and L. Bush. 1985. While the Reagan Administration dozes and scientists vie for glory, the deadly AIDS epidemic has put the entire nation at risk. *Mother Jones.* (April): 32.

Verwoerdt, A. 1966. Defense mechanisms and their management and emotional reactions and their management. In *Communication with the fatally ill,* ed. A. Verwoerdt, 53–91. Springfield, IL: Charles C Thomas, Publisher.

Weinberg, G. 1972. *Society and the healthy homosexual.* New York: St. Martin's Press Inc.

Weisman, A., and W. Worden. 1976. The existential plight in cancer: Significance of the first 100 days. *International Journal of Psychiatry in Medicine* 25: 1–15.

Wortman, C.B. 1983. Social support and the cancer patient: Conceptual and metho-
    dologic issues. *Cancer* 53 (Supplement): 2341.
Young, S. 1986. The exceptional cancer patient support group: Coping with cancer.
    Journal of Holistic Nursing 4: 6–13.

PART II

Long-Term Care Strategy and Management

The Need for a Long-Term Care Strategy

Dennis P. Andrulis

During the first years of the AIDS epidemic, the locus of organized medical care for AIDS patients was almost exclusively the hospital, especially its inpatient unit. As the numbers of infected individuals and the attendant costs of inpatient care escalated and as the manifestations of the epidemic changed, i.e., the identification of many neurological problems and the prolongation of life due to the introduction of new treatments such as azidothymidine (AZT), healthcare providers reassessed the current modes of AIDS service delivery. More importantly, however, a consensus among providers and advocates alike began to emerge: not only was the inpatient bed an inappropriate place to focus healthcare resources, but the needs of people with AIDS extended beyond the hospital walls. Health professionals and concerned individuals clearly realized that they must consider AIDS from the long-term care perspective.

This chapter presents an overview of the placement of people with AIDS outside the hospital. It identifies both the objectives of a long-term care system and the individuals whom such a system is meant to serve. It presents components of an AIDS continuum of care, including the types of services that should be provided in the different settings. Conclusions and implications identify obstacles to developing adequate long-term care for people with AIDS and suggest approaches to overcoming them.

Inpatient Treatment and
Out-of-Hospital Placement

Recognizing that AIDS was becoming one of the major healthcare issues for their memberships, the National Association of Public Hospitals (NAPH) and the Association of American Medical Colleges, Council of Teaching Hospitals (COTH) disseminated a survey to their 465 member hospitals in early 1986. This instrument requested extensive information on the characteristics of AIDS patients, services, and financing during 1985. One hundred sixty-nine institutions, or 42% of the membership responded in detail to the request (Andrulis 1987a, 1987b).

To identify the extent to which public and private teaching institutions were discharging AIDS patients to organized settings, hospitals were asked to cite discharge disposition. As Figure 4-1 shows, the great majority of people with AIDS who were discharged alive (1,600 were deceased at discharge) were sent home without assistance (82% or 4,357 out of 5,325 discharges). Only 5% were placed in a skilled nursing facility or other long-term care setting, and 6% received skilled nursing care at home.

Several factors contribute to the very low placement of the AIDS patients in organized care outside the hospital. Many discharged patients, particularly those in a stage of remission, may not need additional care at that time. Others will have resources available to them. A number of hospitals that may not have coordinated their information internally may have actually placed AIDS patients in organized care but not conveyed that information to the appropriate offices. The NAPH/COTH study found, for instance, that fewer than 25% of the 169 responding hospitals had developed the capacity to monitor and track outpatient utilization by AIDS inpatients during 1985. Still other institutions may have not placed patients directly but may instead have worked through community-based organizations such as the Shanti Project in San Francisco. Even considering these circumstances, the very high proportion of people with AIDS identified as discharged without organized care belies a fundamental lack of posthospital service use.

5,325 live discharges (77% of total patients)

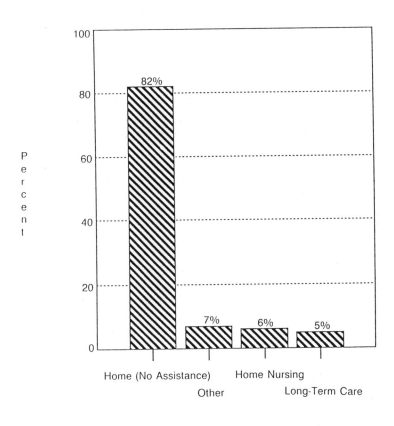

Figure 4-1 Discharge Location for AIDS Patients.

Objectives of an AIDS Long-Term Care System

Incentives to develop, implement, maintain, and enhance long-term care and related support systems for people with AIDS are based on at least three fundamental objectives.

1. Services must be provided which address the spectrum of AIDS patient needs.

2. The use of unnecessary and inappropriate acute care inpatient facilities where costs may be 50-80% higher than nonacute care settings should be reduced to a minimum.

3. Treatment of AIDS patients in their homes or in residential community settings should be emphasized, whenever possible.

Thus, long-term care for people with AIDS must be viewed within the broader context of a continuum of care. Considerations must also include the unique characteristics of this disease such as the life-expectancy of the AIDS patient, the cycles and stages of the illness, and the variations in service intensity required to meet patient needs (Presidential Commission on the Human Immunodeficiency Virus Epidemic 1988).

System Components

Public and private teaching hospitals located in the nation's major urban areas have been struggling at the forefront of the AIDS epidemic for several years. In their capacity as healthcare providers they have identified the following components as integral to any long-term and related support system of care (Presidential Commission on the Human Immunodeficiency Virus Epidemic 1988).

AIDS Prevention, Education, and Assessment

These programs must be put in place for all residents of the community while targeting, in particular, high risk groups. Voluntary testing should be encouraged among those at greatest risk.

Early Intervention with the Healthcare System

Establishing effective outpatient and clinic programs may enable people with AIDS or human immunodeficiency virus (HIV) infection to find treatment without requiring inpatient hospitalization. Moreover, making these service programs one of the cornerstones of care and initial entry points to the healthcare system may help coordinate the service components that are required at later stages of the illness.

Inpatient and Outpatient Hospital Care

A well-integrated system of care would require inpatient treatment only where it is clearly necessary rather than serving as a substitute for other services. Flexibility in design would allow hospitals to treat patients either on special units or in beds throughout the hospitals depending on which approach makes the best use of the institutions' resources. Outpatient care would become the focus of hospital services and would use case managers to coordinate placement out of the hospital.

Nonacute Organized Healthcare Settings

Access to appropriate and adequate subacute care is clearly essential to a successful continuum, enabling patients to obtain care out of the hospital while receiving necessary planned, institution-based treatment. Skilled nursing, intermediate, hospice, and related settings that respond to the needs of AIDS patients must be made available for the ever-increasing number of these individuals who do not require hospitalization but who cannot function in a home without assistance. Comprehensive home-based care can also occur through visiting nurse programs and other supportive entities (e.g., meals on wheels).

Supervised Residential Care

Among the individuals suffering from AIDS are those who may not need the skilled nursing and intermediate care available in organized subacute care settings, but who still require assistance in daily living activities and in monitoring medications. As part of the continuum of care, supervised residential care, including or in conjunction with day care, can ensure that adults and children with AIDS, who do not have a home environment conducive to care, can receive essential support.

Case Management

In many circles, case management (sometimes referred to as services management) has become a commonly used phrase. Nonetheless, the fundamental concepts embodied in case management (assessment, overseeing care and financing, services coordination and monitoring, and planning) must be incorporated into any long-term and related support service system for people with AIDS.

Provider and Community Organization

Execution of an effective continuum of care system cannot be accomplished without the active area-wide participation of communities, their healthcare providers, businesses, and other important sectors. Such involvement with AIDS must include these public and private sector representatives if any new initiative is to be conducted. Providers in particular must work to coordinate and monitor healthcare activities and the needs of people with AIDS through review and advisory groups.

In developing a measured and comprehensive response, communities and their providers must recognize that the population suffering from AIDS and related conditions is not homogeneous. Rather, it is composed of diverse subgroups whose health and social service needs may differ significantly. Thus, a city may have to consider effective interventions for homosexuals, intravenous drug users, women and children, hemophiliacs, bisexuals, the homeless and mentally ill, and persons who may represent many of these characteristics. The nature of AIDS makes it likely that the majority of these people will need some kind of long-term care assistance during the course of their illness.

Development of a Long-Term Care System

The ability to establish and maintain effective systems of care must not be considered as existing in isolation. Rather, several key factors involving the environment within which healthcare providers function significantly influence whether and how long-term care and related services to people with AIDS are delivered (Werdegar et al. 1987).

The following factors represent some fundamental issues to consider in the context of a continuum of care.

Changes in Clinical Manifestations of AIDS

Discoveries concerning the prevalence, length and pattern of infection, and virulence continue to occur with great frequency. New manifestations of the illness may very well require both alteration in services delivery and flexibility to adapt to new clinical directions.

Changes in the AIDS Population

The composition of the AIDS population is not static. As new clinical manifestations are identified, as different areas of the country see more cases, as the AIDS virus affects different risk groups, and as the sheer number of people infected increases, any long-term care and related services initiatives will need reassessment and adjustment.

Identification of New Treatment Protocols

The introduction of new treatments for AIDS that affect the severity, manifestation, longevity of afflicted patients, or other aspects of the illness will alter approaches to service delivery. The best example to date is AZT, which has resulted in a further shift to outpatient healthcare and which will, in all likelihood, trigger a reassessment in long-term care needs related to AIDS.

Impact of Community Attitudes

The concerns of the community about AIDS- and HIV-infected individuals will significantly influence the scope, visibility, and effectiveness of long-term care and related service programs. Where citizens are unwilling to recognize as legitimate the healthcare needs of people with AIDS, realization of innovative or far reaching initiatives will be severely restricted. Conversely, localities that understand that afflicted individuals should be treated with compassion and support will be more likely to finance and otherwise assist in providing appropriate treatment.

Financing

Any existing or proposed program must identify funding sources and assess the likelihood of obtaining and maintaining support. Currently, state and local governments are serving as the major financiers for long-term care, with Medicaid and some demonstration funds from federal and private sources also contributing.

Increasing Dependence on Public Sector Support

Evidence from recent research and from the Healthcare Financing Administration indicates that Medicaid and state and local government support account for substantial if not the major sources of financial assistance for people with AIDS. Moreover, as these individuals exhaust personal resources, lose jobs and private insurance, and live longer, they increase the likelihood of becoming dependent on the public sector. Finally, efforts on the part of private insurers to restrict availability of coverage for HIV-infected individuals will place further reliance on public sources.

Resource Availability

Any AIDS long-term care initiative must continually evaluate the availability of resources to serve afflicted individuals from two perspectives: the physical existence of various settings and providers, and the extent to which those resources are actually appropriate for people with AIDS.

Obstacles

Any effort to develop, implement, or maintain AIDS long-term care strategies is likely to be fraught with problems involving resources, service providers, and the patients themselves. While many of these problems are specific to AIDS, some are inherent to the composition and incentives of the United States healthcare system.

Most clear is the historical lack of financial support for services outside the hospital. Since the current system so strongly encourages inpatient care, many providers are left with little choice: treatment in the hospital or none at all.

The increasing difficulty in finding available alternative care beds and settings is well documented. Now, the AIDS patient is competing with the elderly and other groups for these placements, where fear, costs, and concern for business place those afflicted with AIDS at a severe disadvantage. However, even if placement in these settings were available, their ability to meet the healthcare, social, and support service needs of people with AIDS is open to question.

Finally, subgroups of AIDS patients themselves create major barriers to long-term care. What traditional subacute setting is willing or capable of treating substantial numbers of AIDS people who are homeless, chronically mentally ill, intravenous drug users, or patients with combinations of these characteristics?

Conclusions

As the AIDS epidemic unfolds, the long-term services required by affected individuals are becoming increasingly evident. What lies ahead for AIDS patients seeking a well-coordinated viable system of long-term care is far from clear.

Under the current approach, people with AIDS can expect that unless they have substantial personal and healthcare resources, they will be at the mercy of the same fragmented approach to care faced by other indigent and low income individuals. They can also expect continued difficulty in gaining access to alternate care.

Options to improve the situation are already being proposed or implemented on a limited basis in certain communities. For example, the Robert Wood Johnson Foundation has supported a number of demonstration projects to coordinate care for people with AIDS by using a case management model and community-based organizations. Residential facilities for intravenous drug users such as the Bailey House in New York City and a proposed program in Newark, NJ, begin to address the shelter problems faced by the groups who are hard to serve. New York State is in the process of supporting the development of AIDS centers in hospitals across the state. Such initiatives will include responsibility for assuring that AIDS patients receive all the related medical and supportive care necessary. Moreover, the state is contemplating establishing such centers for alternate care as well, contracting with existing long-term care and related entities to case manage and integrate these services.

These models are just a few of the novel approaches to alternate care being attempted by states and communities. However, the lack of a more widespread effort to develop systems of care attests to three glaring inadequacies: a nonexistent national service policy with regard to AIDS, a dangerously low level of financial support at the federal level for alternate care efforts, and a lack of coordinated involvement among the various public and private sector entities. Without resolution of these barriers, the outlook on and beyond the horizon for those individuals suffering from AIDS in indeed bleak.

References

Andrulis, D.P., et al. 1987a. State Medicaid policies and hospital care for AIDS patients. *Health Affairs* 6: 110–118.
Andrulis, D.P., et al. 1987b. The provision and financing of medical care for AIDS patients in U.S. public and private teaching hospitals. *Journal of the American Medical Association* 258: 1343–1346.
Presidential Commission on the Human Immunodeficiency Virus Epidemic. 1988. Statement of Marc H. Lory, 13 Jan.
Werdegar, D., et al. 1987. AIDS in San Francisco: Status report and plan for fiscal year 1987–88. San Francisco Department of Public Health (Feb., revised Mar.).

CHAPTER 5

Nursing Home Care

Robert C. Marlowe

Acceptance of AIDS patients by nursing homes has been hampered by misconceptions regarding the ability of nursing homes to provide care for such patients. The majority of nursing homes nationwide have decided against admitting individuals solely on the basis of a diagnosis of AIDS. The reasons offered for refusing to care for AIDS patients vary. This chapter discusses a number of concerns regarding the care of AIDS patients in nursing homes and attempts to differentiate between those concerns which are based on fear and those which are legitimate and need attention in order to ensure that all individuals receive appropriate care. Perspectives presented in this chapter are based on experience in the management of a six-facility nursing home chain which has admitted over 35 AIDS and AIDS-related complex (ARC) patients in the past three and one-half years.

Discrimination against AIDS patients is not limited to a refusal to care for individuals falling within the Centers for Disease Control (CDC) definition of AIDS but also includes individuals who have ARC and those who have merely tested positive for exposure to the human immunodeficiency virus (HIV).

Concerns expressed within the industry regarding the care of HIV-positive patients in nursing homes fall into three broad categories: staff, family, and management. The concerns of the family members of staff are considered as part of the concerns of the staff members themselves.

Staff/Staff Family Concerns

The first category, staff and staff family concerns, is effectively characterized by the ultimatum given to some staff members by their spouses: "If you are going to continue to work at that place that takes care of AIDS patients, you don't need to bother coming home." The employee is in the untenable position of having to choose between loyalty to work and loyalty to family. While the employee can not be faulted for choosing family over job, the need for educating the general population regarding AIDS becomes readily apparent.

Nursing homes should not have to shoulder the entire burden of educating the public. This responsibility should rest with the federal and state governments. It is not unreasonable to consider implementation of a nationwide educational program designed to deliver accurate AIDS information to every household in the United States. AIDS education has been incorporated into the school curriculum at the earliest possible grade (Department of Health and Human Services 1986). However, it is imperative that AIDS education programs reach the parents of school children as well. We cannot afford to allow misinformation and panic to dictate public or private action regarding AIDS care.

Health care employees are not immune from the misinformation and hysteria that have developed surrounding AIDS. Any nursing home considering the admission of an HIV-positive patient should take steps to provide complete information about AIDS to all its employees. While the HIV virus does present a small but discrete risk to healthcare workers, it is important that employees not be overwhelmed by irrational fears of contracting AIDS through casual contact with HIV-positive patients.

Initial staff education should begin as soon as possible, and information regarding AIDS should be incorporated into the continuing education programs held at the facility. It is recommended that these programs be conducted with small groups of employees to allow for interaction between the speaker and the employees in attendance. Semiannual updates are not too frequent.

A variety of educational materials are available ranging from cartoon format booklets to videotapes and films (Table 5-1). Infectious disease specialists in private practice or from local universities,

Table 5-1 Educational Resources

New educational materials regarding AIDS are published frequently. Some useful sources include:

Company	Sample Publications
Channing L. Bete, Co., Inc. South Deerfield, MA 01373 (413) 665-7611	Scriptographic booklets on AIDS (cartoon format)
The Public Health Service Centers for Disease Control P.O. Box 6003 Rockville, MD 20850	Various publications available through the Government Printing Office
American Health Consultants 67 Peachtree Park Drive NE Atlanta, GA 30309-1397	*AIDS Alert* and *Common Sense about AIDS* (newsletters)
Atlantic Information Services 1050 17th Street NW, Suite 480 Washington, DC 20036 (20) 775-9008	*AIDS Reference Guide* (two-volume clipping service)
American Healthcare Association 1201 L Street NW Washington, DC 20005 (202) 842-4444	*AIDS and the Nursing Home* and *Provider Magazine* (booklet and monthly magazine)
Commerce Clearing House, Inc. 4025 W. Peterson Avenue Chicago, IL 60646	*AIDS—Employer Rights and Responsibilities* (booklet)
Health Council of Pasco-Pinellas Health Council of West Central Florida 9887 North Gandy Boulevard Suite 200 St. Petersburg, FL 33702-2451 (813) 576-7772	*A Closer Look at AIDS* (free booklet)

and infection control nurses from area hospitals may also serve as speakers at in-service training sessions.

Facilities need to develop a reputation with their staff members for providing accurate information on a timely basis. Employee trust that management is providing accurate information about AIDS is essential in maintaining a rational attitude toward the care of HIV-positive patients.

Facilities must also make sure that their employees have adequate supplies of all materials (gloves, gowns, etc.) necessary to care for AIDS patients. This will address employee fears about not being allowed to take appropriate precautions.

Nursing homes should give serious consideration to purchasing educational materials intended for the public to distribute to the families of staff members. Such materials are available from many of the same sources as materials designed for educating healthcare workers. The key is to maintain an open dialogue with all interested parties.

Patient/Patient Family Concerns

There has been some concern on the part of patients' families regarding the first HIV-positive patients admitted to a nursing home. "Can my mother catch AIDS from that new patient?" is a common question.

Reassuring the family that it is very unlikely that their parent will contract a primarily sexually transmitted disease is usually all that is necessary. Although nursing home patients may be sexually active, there are several reasons why it is doubtful that the typical geriatric patient in a nursing home would become involved in a sexual liaison with an HIV-positive patient. Foremost among these reasons are age differences, differing sexual orientations, and the poor health of HIV-positive persons.

The facility needs to show that its staff is professional and capable of handling HIV-positive and other patients who are difficult to care for. The staff members need training to provide such care, but it is almost as important to make sure that the patients, their families, and the community are aware that the facility provides care of a higher quality than the public general perceives as typical for nursing homes.

Reassurance, both about AIDS and about the competence level of the staff may take the form of one-on-one conferences with the administrator or medical director, small group meetings, or educational brochures about AIDS. AIDS is an ideal topic for presentation at family support groups and resident council meetings. A combination of different approaches seems to be the most effective way to communicate accurate information to patients and their families.

The reaction of the community seems to be less intense toward the admission of HIV-positive patients to existing nursing homes than it is to the prospect of having a separate AIDS facility or unit. The community response to admitting patients has been mixed but mild compared to the reaction in one community when a facility announced that it was going to set up an AIDS unit. The facility was almost immediately beset by neighbors carrying picket signs. Local television crews and newspaper photographers made certain that everyone in the area knew that the idea of AIDS patients in the neighborhood was not a welcome one.

This type of reaction may well be one of the best reasons for placing HIV-positive patients into existing nursing facilities (mainstreaming) rather than trying to set up special units. Furthermore, in most locations there are not enough HIV-positive patients needing nursing home care to justify the construction of a special unit or facility. Problems associated with mainstreaming HIV-positive patients center on the acceptance of these patients by facilities that historically have not had to deal with any type of infectious disease or with individuals labeled as outcasts by society. Most of these problems have the potential to exist regardless of whether the patient is in an existing facility or a special unit.

Managerial Concerns

Management should have a number of concerns regarding the care of HIV-positive patients in the nursing home. Unfortunately, an irrational fear of AIDS seems to be the overriding one. It would be more appropriate for nursing home administrators to address care requirements, costs, media exposure, Workers' Compensation coverage, employees at risk, and health and general liability insurance coverage when preparing to care for HIV-positive patients.

Ability to Provide Care

Foremost among these concerns is whether or not the personnel of a nursing home are capable of providing the care required by HIV-positive patients. Since the CDC recommends that hospitals and nursing homes institute "Universal Precautions" for exposure to blood and body fluids (Centers for Disease Control 1985), all nursing homes should train their staff members to observe blood and body fluid precautions with *all* patients; and since these are the same precautions recommended by the CDC when caring for HIV-infected individuals, it should follow that all facilities should be capable of instituting and maintaining adherence to the proper infection control procedures.

As part of the move toward "Universal Precautions," facilities will see an increase in the utilization of gloves, gowns, and other disposable items. However, this will occur regardless of whether or not HIV-positive patients are admitted. Current spot shortages of gloves would seem to indicate that healthcare providers are beginning to implement "Universal Precautions."

The disposal of syringes and other sharps is a critical area of concern. Facility staff members need training in the proper method of disposing of these implements. Most nurses and others who use needles and syringes learned in school to recap syringe needles. It is imperative that these individuals be retrained to refrain from this extremely risky practice. The large majority of incidents where healthcare workers have potentially exposed themselves to HIV have been needlestick injuries, and they are avoidable by following proper disposal procedures (Centers for Disease Control 1987).

Arrangements for the disposal of infective waste should provide for the transport of such materials to a neighboring hospital or some other location equipped with an incinerator. There is no epidemiological evidence that general nursing home waste is any more infective than residential waste, and therefore it is *not* necessary to incinerate everything coming out of a facility utilizing universal precautions (American Healthcare Association 1987).

Some HIV-positive patients have difficulty swallowing, and therefore a number of small meals may better suit these individuals than the typical three-meal routine found in nursing homes. This is not a major problem but does require some adjustment on the part of the dietary staff.

Facilities face, for the first time, the situation of a patient receiving an experimental drug. This may necessitate applying for and receiving special approval from the state pharmacy and nursing home licensing agencies for the use of experimental drugs within the facility. New facility policies and procedures are needed regarding the protocol for use of experimental drugs.

HIV-positive patients present some rather unique challenges to the social service and activities staff. These patients are typically much younger than the average nursing home patient, and their interests tend to be different. An activities program consisting primarily of bingo, quilting, crafts, and other activities geared for elderly female patients will no longer be adequate when young HIV-positive patients are admitted to the facility. Special efforts are required to develop and offer activities that will be of interest to relatively young male patients. Because the number of patients involved is likely to be small, the Activities Director can solicit suggestions regarding activities of interest directly from the HIV-positive patients. AIDS patients may isolate themselves from the other patients, and it is incumbent upon the social service and activities staff members to make a special effort to get them involved and socializing with other patients and staff members.

Difficulties in finding nursing homes willing to accept HIV-positive patients have resulted in a number of these patients being physically isolated from what remains of their support network due to their admission to a facility some distance from home. Contact with a local AIDS support group can provide these patients with a new network. Where such groups are not available, the social service designee should be making an extra effort to find people willing to visit and spend extra time with an HIV-positive patient.

One final element of care provision that has proven to be difficult to arrange is physician and dental services. Unfortunately, there are physicians who will drop a patient when they learn that he or she carries HIV; therefore, nursing homes need to maintain a close relationship with physicians willing to take such patients.

There has also been reluctance on the part of dentists to provide care to HIV-positive patients. Representatives of the Florida Dental Association addressed the AIDS Workshop of the Florida Statewide Health Council on November 19, 1987, to object to the Council's recommendation that healthcare providers refusing to care for AIDS patients be delicensed. Further education of dental professionals should improve access for HIV-positive patients in the future, but patients need care now.

It is within the technical expertise level of most nursing homes to provide care to HIV-positive patients. The infection control measures required are well within the range of measures required by the federal government of all facilities participating in the Medicare, Medicaid, or Veterans Administration nursing home programs (Healthcare Financing Administration 1987). The remaining management concerns revolve around the costs and legal implications of providing care to HIV-positive patients.

Costs

The ability of a facility to provide care at a cost that will allow it to remain financially sound is a critical concern of every manager. The additional direct care expenses involved in caring for HIV-positive patients fall in two broad categories: the costs of disposable items, and the cost of providing for patients who require more direct care than other patients.

The first of these—the costs associated with the use of disposable items—should be moot since facilities should be instituting "Universal Precautions" anyway. The larger problem is that these costs will apply not just to HIV-positive patients, but to all patients within the facility. State Medicaid programs pay for a significant portion of nursing home costs nationwide, and those programs need to recognize that the adoption of universal precautions is going to have a measurable impact on the cost of providing care to nursing home patients. It is important for nursing home administrators to make sure that the state legislatures are aware of this increase in cost when setting Medicaid budgets.

The second problem of the direct patient care needs requires closer attention. Many HIV-positive patients have been extremely sick and have required significant nursing time to care for their various medical problems. This time requirement appears to be related to the non-HIV-associated medical problems rather than the HIV infection itself. This may not be as significant a problem for facilities accustomed to caring for ventilator-dependent and other high-care patients, but it will be a problem for facilities accustomed to caring for a patient population made up predominantly of intermediate or custodial care patients.

It would be valuable to conduct a large scale study comparing the cost of maintaining HIV-positive patients in nursing homes with the cost of maintaining more typical geriatric patients in the same facilities.

Media Exposure

It is probably a gross understatement to say that most nursing home administrators would rather not be at the center of media attention, particularly when it involves sensationalism regarding the staff reaction to the admission of AIDS patients. The administrator needs to try to keep the reporting as factual as possible without violating the patients' right to privacy in the process. Because nursing homes are relatively small entities, it is impossible to admit an atypical patient without virtually the whole staff knowing about it within minutes. Training staff members about patient confidentiality helps, but all it takes is one person calling the local media to get things rolling. The administrator needs to be ready to handle such occurrences in a way that will avoid exposing the facility to adverse publicity and possible legal actions.

Workers' Compensation Concerns

The most significant problem in the area of Workers' Compensation is proving that an employee acquired an HIV infection as a result of exposure on the job and not as a result of his or her extracurricular activities. Workers' Compensation laws vary from state to state. In Florida, for instance, the burden lies with the employer to prove that an injury was *not* received on the job.

Some individuals will refuse to admit to any high risk activity because of the social stigmas associated with some of the practices that result in exposure to HIV. It would certainly be tempting to blame a positive test result on an incident at work rather than admitting to cheating on one's spouse, engaging in homosexual activities, or using illegal drugs.

It is imperative that nursing homes track carefully any incident involving needlestick injuries and other similar potential exposures to HIV-infected blood. Testing of the employee immediately and at the six-week, three-month, six-month, and one-year anniversaries of the incident is appropriate (Centers for Disease Control 1985). Employees involved in such incidents need counseling about safeguards to prevent potential transmission of the virus until the receipt of test results.

Nursing homes need to develop policies regarding the testing of patients of unknown HIV status in the event of such an incident. A negative test result for the patient's blood will reassure the employee long before he or she could otherwise complete the test sequence. It should be apparent that the facility would have to receive informed consent from the patient before testing for the virus.

There is also the question of how many employees are already at risk. As with any large organization, it is almost certain that there are employees who are in high risk groups. Individuals falling within one or more of the identified risk groups are far more likely to seroconvert as a result of participation in a high risk activity than from exposure on the job.

The availability of Workers' Compensation, group health, and general liability insurance has been of concern to some administrators. It has been our experience that providing care to HIV-positive patients has had absolutely no impact on either the availability or cost of such insurance.

There is a concern that a facility accepting HIV-positive patients will not be able to recruit and retain staff members. Thorough education of staff members will serve to minimize turnover related to a decision to admit HIV-positive patients. It is reassuring to know that employees quitting their jobs because of the admission of AIDS patients will not be able to collect unemployment compensation, as such a resignation is not for "good cause" (Cooper v. Bear Creek Nursing Center 1985). Properly handled, it is possible for the admission of HIV-positive patients to become routine and to result in no disruption of the facility.

In order to put into perspective the question of whether or not nursing homes should care for HIV-positive patients, we should address the question of what to do with an employee or job applicant who has tested positive for the virus. There is a growing body of case law suggesting that it is illegal to discriminate against individuals who either have AIDS or who have tested positive for HIV. Nursing homes need to develop policies and procedures for dealing with these employees. From a management perspective, simply identifying such individuals and confirming that the case is not job related is extremely important. Of course, any measures used for identifying HIV-positive employees must ensure that all information regarding the test status remains confidential. Routine testing of employees and job applicants is not appropriate. There are no positions within a nursing home setting where a negative HIV status could be considered a bona fide occupational qualification.

Development of case law in the employment area may render moot the whole question of whether or not a facility should accept HIV-positive patients. An institution prohibited by law from discriminating against employees on the basis of being HIV-seropositive is going to be hard pressed to justify discriminating against HIV-seropositive clients.

Conclusions

It should be clear that nursing homes have a moral and legal responsibility to provide care for HIV-positive patients, that nursing homes either have or should have the technical expertise to care for them, and that none of the problems associated with the care of HIV-positive patients in a nursing home setting is insurmountable.

Recent case law, state legislation, and changes in interpretation of existing law by the federal government make it clear that HIV-positive patients will be considered handicapped under various state and federal laws and therefore cannot be discriminated against in the provision of government-funded services.

Nursing homes are capable of taking the appropriate precautions for dealing with HIV-positive patients. Adherence to "Universal Precautions" for exposure to blood and body fluids render this issue moot.

Finally, the other problems associated with the care of these patients can be minimized through the establishment of an ongoing education program for staff, patients, and their families.

References

American Healthcare Association. 1987. *AIDS and the nursing home.* Dec.: 44

Centers for Disease Control. 1985. Recommendations for preventing transmission of infection with human T-lymphotropic virus type III / lymphadenopathy associated virus in the workplace. *Morbidity and Mortality Weekly Report* 34: 681–685, 691–694.

Centers for Disease Control. 1987. Recommendations for prevention of HIV transmission in health-care settings. *Morbidity and Mortality Weekly Report.* 36 (Supplement): 4S–6S.

Department of Health and Human Services. 1986. *Surgeon General's Report on acquired immune deficiency syndrome.* Washington, D.C.: Government Printing Office.

Healthcare Financing Administration. 1987. *Code of Federal Regulations* (Title 42): Section 405.1135. Washington, D.C.: Government Printing Office.

CHAPTER 6

Hospice Care

Monica Adams Koshuta

The provision of long-term care for persons with AIDS during the chronic and terminal stage of the disease is a challenging issue that the healthcare system must confront. Since October, 1986, a limited number of persons with AIDS have participated in the azidothymidine (AZT) drug protocols and have experienced a prolongation of life by approximately six months. Quality care during this period of chronicity has been uncertain and in some cases unavailable. Consequently, the healthcare system is now confronted with providing care outside an acute care facility for an extended period of time. This chapter describes how one long-term care institution provides care for patients who have a limited prognosis and who have their needs met through a hospice. The chapter also includes the steps used before and during the implementation of the services for AIDS patients at Hospice of Washington, a program of the Washington Home which is a long-term care facility located in the District of Columbia and which was one of the first hospice programs in the United States to provide inpatient care for patients with AIDS.

Description of the Hospice Program

Hospice of Washington is a comprehensive Medicare facility which has provided services for terminally ill residents of metropolitan Washington, D.C. for the past 10 years in an inpatient unit at The Washington Home. In 1986, the implementation of a hospice home care program made Hospice of Washington the first comprehensive hospice in the area.

71

The inpatient facility is a nine-bed unit located on one of the long-term care wings of The Washington Home. There is no physical barrier separating the unit from the rest of the home. Only a sign identifies the hospice area, serving as a welcome notice but also advising all visitors to check with the hospice staff before entering. Because confidentiality is important, no patient names are visible, assuring them of privacy and control during their time in the hospice.

Although Hospice of Washington is part of a long-term care facility, it is separate and distinct with its own administration and staff. Dietary, housekeeping, engineering, and financial services are provided by the long-term care staff. Nursing, social work, chaplaincy, admissions, volunteers, coordinators, and the administrator are hospice staff, while medical services are provided by the geriatric team that serves long-term care patients as well. One of the long-term care physicians serves as the medical director of the hospice.

The needs of the nine hospice patients are met by two registered nurses on each shift, supplemented by a nursing assistant on the day shift, a social worker, volunteers for 12 to 15 hours a day, and the chaplain for 20 hours a week. Families and friends may visit the patients 24 hours a day and may spend the night if they choose. Patients and families are involved in decision making and are encouraged to participate in planning and implementation of care.

The Hospice Concept

Hospice is a concept of care; it is not a particular place or institution. Eighty percent of hospice care is provided in the patient's home, however, when a patient's condition warrants more intensive care, inpatient care is available. Most hospice programs provide both types of care. For persons with AIDS, hospice care in the privacy of their homes is usually appropriate until they require the services of professional nursing staff on an inpatient basis. The decision for inpatient hospice care is made by the patient, family or significant other, and the physician.

The hospice philosophy views death as a realistic event but supports life to its fullest until death. A hospice does nothing to shorten life. Its goal is to provide palliative or comfort care. Patients are encouraged to live their remaining days as they choose. Patients are viewed as members of a social unit. Consequently, the patient and family or significant others become the unit of care and are provided with support and assistance in coming to grips with the patient's prognosis and death. Hospice care is planned from a holistic viewpoint. In addition to the patient's physiological needs, the patient's emotional, social, and spiritual requirements are considered as well. This holistic approach provides support for the patients as they strive to cope with the impending loss over which they have no control.

Hospice care is provided by a multidisciplinary team directed by a physician including nursing, social work, pastoral counseling, adjunctive therapies, and volunteer services as well. Hospice home care provides for a team member to be on call 24 hours a day, 7 days a week. Bereavement care is available to the survivors for 13 months following the death of the patient, assisting family members and significant others to resolve their grief (Amenta 1986).

Commitment

All healthcare providers recognize their responsibility to provide quality service. The current challenge is making a commitment to provide this quality care to persons with AIDS. In addition to making the commitment, the organization must also overcome many barriers in already operating programs, including the existing policy of not providing services or admitting patients with infectious or communicable diseases; fear of contracting the disease; inadequate reimbursement; fear of loss of referrals; and problems with existing patients, clients, or residents.

In addition, AIDS is a disease associated with the American taboos of homosexuality, drugs, and death. Any one of these issues alone could be an insurmountable force, and their combination provides a challenge even to the most experienced and competent caregivers and administrators.

Commitment to the provision of care for AIDS clients involves seeking input from staff, administration, and the governing body of the organization. Consequently, special meetings are needed for each level. The initial sessions should be a time of dialogue and an opportunity for the participants to express their doubts and concerns. The importance of active listening by educators and administrators should not be underestimated. These meetings need to allow ample time for employees not only to express their concerns, their doubts and their fears but also to work through their ambivalent feelings about providing care for these patients. The sessions should be conducted in a nonthreatening informal manner.

It is during this type of interaction that an assessment can be made about the level of education and training required to assist staff members in understanding the long-term care needs of persons with AIDS. The administration needs to be aware that this education and training may be time consuming and costly, therefore adequate resources are essential. Training must be provided for all . There is as much misinformation as there is information about this disease, and healthcare agencies have a responsibility to provide education that will deal with employee concerns and fears.

The first fear that must be addressed is the transmissibility of AIDS. There has been and will continue to be fear among the healthcare providers of contracting the disease. To dispel this fear, the information provided must be based on the facts that are available from reliable sources such as the Centers for Disease Control, the National Institutes of Health, as well as local, state, and federal public health departments. Persons with AIDS are frequently willing to participate in these training programs. Many audiovisual resources are also available at little or no cost, for example, local Red Cross and public health offices have pamphlets, often available in multiple languages.

The second most common fear is that of confronting death. This is not surprising since we live in a society that depicts death as the enemy. Consequently, caregivers may have difficulty in dealing with persons who are facing the final phase of living and their eventual death. Although education on the care of the person with AIDS should emphasize life, death must be viewed as the realistic outcome, and these patients should not feel abandoned during the terminal stage of their illness.

Care needs increase for the patient and family and significant others during this final stage—the dying process. Staffing needs to be adjusted to accommodate these escalated needs to prevent burnout among the caregivers.

The final fear is that of the populations having the greatest numbers of AIDS cases—homosexual or bisexual males and intravenous drug users. Caregivers, for their own personal reasons, may be ambivalent about working with or providing care to these patients. They need time and support to work through these feelings and to digest the factual information about the disease. Support for the staff and sensitivity to their feelings are imperative if any new program is to be successful.

Implementation

The success or failure of implementing a program that provides care and support for persons with AIDS depends on a staff that understands the disease process itself and also the care that is required. Because most of the patients seeking long-term services will have a limited prognosis, a small staff may be adequate. Admissions should be restricted to a few patients until the staff feels comfortable with the level, quality, and quantity of care.

Symptom Management and Level of Care

The level of care for patients with AIDS depends on their stage of the disease process. Symptom management begins with the initial assessment and continues throughout the course of the illness. Long-term symptom control is a crucial element if these patients are to have comfort and quality in their lives. Rapid changes in both their physical and mental status are not unusual as the disease progresses. The physiological problems of AIDS patients usually include fever, marked weight loss, severe diarrhea, and night sweats. According to results of several studies reported in the *American Journal of Nursing* (Staff 1987), physical care needs were 28-41% higher for patients with AIDS than for other medical patients. Staffing patterns need adjustment to meet this increased demand.

Another disturbing symptom for the patient with AIDS is dementia which usually begins with impaired memory and difficulties in concentration. As the disease progresses either insidiously or overtly, the dementia may present with other symptoms including incontinence of bowel and bladder and weakness or the inability to move one or more extremities. This weakness commonly affects the lower extremities and interferes with the patient's ability to walk. In addition, patients may experience dysfunctioning of the nervous system and varying intensities of sensitivity to touch or pain. Aphasia or the loss of the ability to articulate speech is another common problem that may be a result of the dementia.

The dementia causes cognitive impairment, and patients may find themselves unable to provide adequate information to the caregiver about their pain and discomfort. Frequently, these patients benefit from analgesia, even though they have not been able to verbalize their discomfort; therefore nonverbal communication indicative of pain needs to be considered in the assessment process.

Psychosocial and spiritual pain may be of a greater intensity than the physical pain and should be addressed by the appropriate members of the staff. Counseling and active listening skills are crucial. Time should be provided for the patient to express feelings about his fear of death. The patient and family and significant others may be going through the painful process of anticipatory grief. Providing support in their grieving adds to the time required on the part of the staff.

Spiritual needs are often more pressing than the need for religion at time of approaching death although some spiritual needs may be met through religion. The staff should be aware of the individualistic nature of these needs among their AIDS patients.

Hydration and nutrition may be problematic because of a decrease in appetite accompanied by diarrhea. Nutritional assessments should outline the patient's food preferences and eating habits. Frequent small feedings and commercially prepared dietary supplements may provide additional intake to help combat or prevent these problems.

The elements of compassion, kindness, and gentleness should be integrated with clinical competency to achieve optimal management of AIDS symptoms. This type of care will provide an atmosphere that enables patients to have a quality life.

Support for the Caregivers

Healthcare organizations recognize that they cannot meet the continual emotional support for patients and families or significant others without addressing the issue of staff stress. Working with terminally ill patients requires not only special training but also adequate support for the staff members themselves. The administration needs to monitor their emotional responses to the repeated losses and establish formal and informal support groups which provide an environment for caregivers to express their feelings and frustrations. Attendance of staff members at memorial services or funerals can help them terminate their emotional ties with patients and families or significant others. Institutional memorial services which remember those who have died are important as they provide another outlet for the staff and have a therapeutic effect on their response to repeated loss (Green 1984).

Concerns of the Provider

There is a potential negative impact which an organization or agency considering the admission of AIDS patients must consider. The following questions are a few that will be encountered. Will acceptance of AIDS patients create a negative image in the community? Will future revenue decrease if caring for AIDS patients has a negative effect on referrals or if the number of clients decreases? Will employees resign? Is it worth taking the risk?

Hospice of Washington confronted these concerns cautiously and with sensitivity to all the populations involved. Education inside the institution as well as involvement in community education were the most important components in addressing them. Education was provided for all levels of employees before the admission of the first patient, and this education is ongoing. Not one staff member has resigned, and Hospice of Washington has witnessed little or no impact on the number of admissions. The admission policy remains unchanged and states that "All terminally ill patients who meet the admission criteria for hospice care will be assessed and admitted accordingly." These criteria include a diagnosis of a terminal illness with a limited prognosis measured in months, curative therapy is not indicated, and the patient is aware of his/her diagnosis and understands the palliative care provided by the hospice and signs a consent for hospice care.

Conclusions

In the past, our healthcare system has met the challenges of tuberculosis, cancer, and polio. It must now confront the challenging issue of providing long-term care services for persons with AIDS. Long-term care providers must recognize the dire need for high quality care and must participate with other providers to achieve the goal of adequate long-term services for the increasing number of terminally ill persons with AIDS. We must be understanding rather than critical or judgmental as efforts continue to deal with the serious and challenging problems associated with AIDS.

References

Amenta, M.O. 1986. The hospice movement. *In Nursing care of the terminally ill*, ed. M.O. Amenta and N. Bohnet, 49–64. Boston: Little, Brown & Co. Inc.

Green, M. 1984. Roles of health professionals and institutions. *In Bereavement: Reactions, consequences and care*, ed. M. Osterweis, F. Solomon, and M. Green, 215–236. Washington, D.C.: National Academy Press.

Staff. 1987. AIDS patients need more nursing time. *American Journal of Nursing* 87: 1540–1542.

CHAPTER 7

The Consumer's Perspective: Matching Patient Needs with Service Capacity

Ann Wyatt

The challenge of the AIDS epidemic highlights the inadequacies and limitations of long-term care in this country. At the same time, the challenge points to the potential that long-term care has to offer people in need of its services.

Because AIDS is so new and so complex in its various manifestations, most of the care provided to people with the disease has, until now, been given in acute care settings. Home care has also been widely available in some locations, but institutional long-term care services have been almost totally unavailable. This chapter will examine the necessity of matching patient needs with the capabilities of various long-term care settings.

Barriers to Long-Term Care in Nursing Homes

There are several issues which have complicated the question of how to make institutional long-term care accessible to people with AIDS. These include concerns about infection control; anxiety over opening up institutions which have traditionally served the elderly to those who have a history of drug use and who are openly gay; questions about the potentially sophisticated and more intensive care requirements; concerns about the adequacy of reimbursement; and not least, the episodic nature of the disease itself.

Obviously, infection control is something which ought not to be new to nursing homes because there are many infections prevalent in such facilities. The fact that nursing homes should have effective infection control programs does not mean that they do, of course, but neither is it an unreasonable expectation. In any case, a home with an existing program that works effectively to control infection should be able to manage control of the human immunodeficiency virus (HIV) as well.

When AIDS patients are known to be homosexual or to have a history of substance abuse there are likely to be some conflicts of life-style with the staff and residents of a nursing home. However, it is incorrect to assume that conflict has been unknown in such settings, for there are often great differences in life-styles among residents and between residents and staff. Behavioral problems, dementia, and mental illness also contribute to the potential for such conflict in nursing homes. Most of all, the tension between the needs of individuals and the requirements of institutions creates conflict which is always present to some degree. What is essential is that there are mechanisms in place to address these problems appropriately and effectively, permitting the institution to define its own limits in particular situations given particular patient populations. Latitude should be extended to those people with AIDS as it is now extended to elderly people.

While it is true that nursing homes have had very little experience in providing care to those who abuse drugs, the more basic problem is that the medical community in general has not advanced very far in providing healthcare to this population. Continued substance abuse in a long-term care setting can have a greater impact, however, than in a hospital because of the differences in lengths of stay and in the acuity of illness.

The institution does, of course, have a responsibility to educate its staff members properly about AIDS and to help them contend with their fears of the disease and also of the people who have been primarily affected by it thus far. It is also responsible for setting clear guidelines for the standards of care and behavior that will be expected of its staff with regard to all patients, whether or not they have AIDS. In addition, institutions have a critical role to play in educating other patients, their relatives and families, and the community at large.

Because AIDS is complex and unpredictable, more than the usual level of sophistication is required of a nursing home that is providing care to AIDS patients. Some of this can be offset by close ties to an acute care facility with AIDS expertise, but the nursing home itself will still have to make some adjustments. These adjustments could include but are not limited to monitoring highly toxic experimental drugs, case management of a patient with several simultaneous infections, and the ability to respond to abrupt and critical changes in clinical status. As can be seen from these examples, the intensity of care required by AIDS patients is often greater than that required by more typical nursing home residents. Clearly, not every nursing home has the capacity for providing such sophisticated care, nor is every nursing home going to have or be able to develop a close working relationship with an acute care hospital experienced in the care of people with AIDS.

Obviously, a home's capacity for providing care is related to the issue of adequate reimbursement; to some extent, the question of reimbursement in turn rests on how many AIDS patients are being cared for in a particular setting. Although any given patient may require an especially intense level of care, the effect of this need on the nursing home as a whole will depend on the overall case mix of patients in the home and on what the average demands on the home's resources are. It is also true, however, that caring for a number of people with AIDS in one setting will usually be more resource-intensive and cost more than caring for a similar sized group of more typical patients. AIDS patients will often not only have more complicated and intensive medical and nursing needs, but extensive psychosocial requirements as well. While these kinds of needs can usually be attended to over time for the more typical patient, this is not usually true for AIDS patients. They often have complicated social situations that result from an impending early death frequently accompanied by guilt and the stigma of the disease itself. Dealing with such complex problems, including work with friends and families, in which is usually a short time frame places enormous demands on social work, psychological, and psychiatric services.

Medical Appropriateness

The discussion so far has focused primarily on what is required of institutions when they care for people with AIDS, but perhaps the more problematic issue is the episodic nature of the disease itself. Long-term care institutions typically care for people who are admitted either because they need a period of rehabilitation or because they are in a period of fairly slow and predictable decline. People with AIDS, on the other hand, have episodes of illness which tend to be erratic. In between these episodes, the patients can be well for long periods of time during which they may not need any care at all. It can happen that the various infections to which AIDS patients are eventually subject so invade the body that functioning becomes greatly impaired and the course of the illness becomes more steadily and predictably downhill. Even then, a patient may continue to experience new episodes of infection which, if the patient wishes, could require diagnostic and treatment procedures that are not available in a nursing home. Because AIDS is episodic in these ways, planning for a continuum of long-term care can be very difficult.

In fact, medically there is no clearly defined point at which it could be said to be appropriate to refer someone with AIDS to a long-term care setting. The need for placement occurs for people with AIDS as it does for the older people who are the primary consumers of long-term care services—largely as a result of the relationship between functional disability, social circumstances, and resource availability. Virtually anyone can be and is cared for in the home setting if their financial resources are in place and if a friend or family member is available to help give care.

What further complicates the issue of medical appropriateness for long-term care is that many, if not most, AIDS patients choose to continue receiving aggressive treatment throughout most of their illness. Even at a point late in the disease process when many overriding functional incapacities may have developed, new episodes of infection can occur. Given the sophistication of the disease and the resulting diagnostic and treatment requirements, many nursing homes will find it difficult to meet these needs.

Alternatively, palliative care is often not readily available in many nursing homes, where it is not uncommon for someone near death to be sent to the hospital. Palliative care is, of course, available in hospice settings, but in general, nursing homes have less experience with responding to the needs of someone in the terminal stage of a difficult and often painful illness.

The Traditional Role of Nursing Homes

In essence, then, although people with AIDS may in fact need long-term care, it cannot be assumed that every long-term care institution is equipped to provide the kind of care these patients may require. This is extremely important, because ignoring these concerns could result in a de facto denial of appropriate care so that AIDS patients would be sent to a long-term care facility on the assumption that such facilities are all equally able to respond appropriately and effectively.

In fact, throughout most of their history, nursing homes have frequently been used to solve the problem of where to put people who have nowhere else to go. Nursing homes house not only older people who are either too frail or too ill to care for themselves, but also people (usually older) who have mental retardation, mental illness, alcoholism, and Alzheimer's disease. This tendency has resulted in the blurring of their care needs, since very few homes have developed the capacity to respond to the specific treatment requirements of each target population.

Compounding the problem even more is that nursing homes have existed significantly apart from the attention of the medical community and from the interest of the neighborhoods in which they are located. While this has begun to change over the past several years, and of course, has not been true for all homes, it has been so for the majority.

Ironically, the lesson this isolation teaches is that wherever possible, the creation of separate facilities for the care of people with AIDS should be avoided. As difficult as it has been over the years to bring the care of older people in nursing homes more into the mainstream, it would be even more difficult to do so with AIDS facilities because of the stigma attached to the disease. Instead, energy should be directed to continuing the gradual progress that has been made over the years to strengthen the ties of long-term care settings to the rest of the medical world.

In addition, as nursing homes have steadily carved out a more accepted and significant role within society, they have also begun to upgrade the care they provide more successfully. This has not been an easy or a painless process. There is inherent tension between the institutions which desire to run smoothly and efficiently and the residents who need and want to retain as much autonomy as possible over the decisions about their care and the daily routine of their lives.

Need for Autonomy

Unlike hospitals, long-term care institutions are much more than settings where nursing and medical care is provided. For most of the people who reside there, they are home as well. This means that philosophically and conceptually, the institutions are supposed to address the needs of the whole person not just that part which is sick. It is important to make the distinction that long-term care institutions cannot and should not be asked to meet all the needs of the people who live there, but they must address them, in the sense of acknowledging their importance. The only real way to do so is to promote throughout the institution the attitude that autonomy, self-sufficiency, and the opportunity for retaining decisions for one's life are essential for a resident's social and emotional health. Such autonomy extends from decisions about medical treatment to the myriad of small activities which make up a day such as when to get up, what to wear, what to eat, which activity to attend (if any), and which book to read. Clearly, in an institutional setting, a patient cannot have unlimited options for such decisions, but the best institutions are those which maximize these options to the fullest possible extent. Regardless of whether a patient can move easily about the institution or is bed bound, it is in the activities of everyday life that autonomy exists most fundamentally.

Usually, institutions are not very good at either acknowledging or promoting the personal autonomy of their residents. Since older people are disenfranchised in so many other aspects of life, the fact that this occurs as much as it does in institutions has not been as noticeable as it might be otherwise. However, most AIDS patients are young, as are their families and friends, and for them the lack of autonomy is likely to be more noticeable and therefore will present more of a challenge to the institutions charged with their care.

Community Involvement

One of the most effective ways for institutions to widen and make more "normal" the world of those who reside there is to seek and promote actively wide ranging roles for volunteers and community members within the institution. This is the surest and best way of appealing to the diverse interests and needs of the residents. Such an effort will not only enrich the lives of all involved, but it can also help dispel the fear and anxiety in communities about people who have AIDS.

Community involvement is also the best way to assure an activities program which is prepared to respond to some of the additional interests which younger people may have. A patient in a long-term care institution, even someone who is fairly ill, does not have very much of the day taken up with care needs, and time is all too often a very heavy burden. This is the particular challenge of an activities program in a long-term care setting and certainly would continue to be so in a setting with AIDS patients.

Targeted Services

Given the limitations of long-term care settings which have been described here, it is not reasonable to expect all nursing homes to care effectively for the full spectrum of extended care needs that AIDS patients may have.

For those patients who require extended care but wish to continue receiving aggressive treatment, processes should be developed to identify those homes which are capable of providing such care. Crucial to such a capacity will be the strength of a nursing home's ties to an acute care facility with AIDS expertise. Probably the most effective way of enhancing a nursing home's ability to provide care to AIDS patients with continuing treatment needs is to select homes which can set aside a group (a floor or a wing) of beds for AIDS patients. In this way, appropriate resources (such as more intensive nursing, consultation services of an infectious disease physician) can be developed and concentrated more effectively, thus permitting a more sophisticated and coordinated approach.

Palliative care, on the other hand, may not require the same degree of acute care back-up and may be easier for less sophisticated homes to provide to a few patients at a time. It will be extremely important, however, for both hospitals and nursing homes caring for AIDS patients to have clearly articulated "Do Not Resuscitate" (DNR) policies and procedures. This point cannot be emphasized enough, since it is central to the task of matching the needs of patients with the capacities of long-term care institutions. Furthermore, although most hospitals are not accustomed to providing long-term care services, for some patients who are close to death it may be more appropriate to keep them there rather than to send them to another setting. It is often not possible to predict when death is near with AIDS patients, but when it is possible to do so, it may be more humane to let them die in what will have become familiar surroundings. Ultimately, it may also be a better use of limited resources.

The hardest extended care problem to solve, however, results from the episodic nature of AIDS. Even if nursing homes (including intermediate care facilities) enhance their programs appropriately, they are not very flexible in the amount of care they can provide, and they are inappropriate and constraining when someone is in a state of recovery and has limited or no care needs. The alternative is all too often that some patients will literally experience a kind of revolving door scenario in which they go back and forth among various levels of care.

Home care is, in fact, the single most flexible service for those with extended care needs. Literally every level of care, from none to hospice and skilled nursing care, can be provided in a home setting, with adjustments made fairly quickly and relatively easily. Home care agencies need to develop many of the capacities cited above for nursing homes, but there are already many precedents for this since home care has, to date, been the primary mode of providing long-term services to people with AIDS. The problem of recruiting and retaining an adequate number of home care personnel should not be minimized, however, but this is a problem for home care in general, not merely with home care for AIDS patients. Of course, people must first have a home where care can be provided, and unfortunately, homelessness is a major factor with those affected by AIDS as it is with other segments of society.

Home care cannot be provided effectively to people whose dementia has progressed to the point where they are unable to be self-directing, and who have no friend or relative able to take on this role. This means that one of the indicators for institutional placement of AIDS patients is dementia, just as is the case with older people. It is possible to have a significant amount of dementia with few or no other symptoms, and institutions need to have the flexibility to take this into account.

The funding streams which are available for extended care tend to be limited to institutions which are organized around a medical model. This means that they have not only limited flexibility in the levels of care they can offer in any one setting, but they are also limited in the degree to which they can respond to the patient as an individual who has more than medical needs. In contrast, any settings which are considered someone's home (including some specialized housing projects and some adult home-type residences) have the potential for more flexibility in both of these areas.

Receiving services at home can mean that someone becomes very isolated, of course, but the person is usually in a much better position to retain control over his or her own daily life. The level of care actually provided can also vary greatly, depending primarily on what a given locale is prepared to offer. For congregate living settings (such as adult homes) where extensive home care can be brought in on an as-needed basis, the concern is understandably raised that the setting is essentially operating as an unlicensed healthcare facility. This concern assumes inadequacies in the way that home care services are monitored; a process that is never easy. However, consideration should be given to enhanced and perhaps more creative ways of monitoring such care for people with AIDS and for others as well.

Conclusions

As treatments continue to be developed which extend the life span of those with AIDS, more and more people who are symptomatic will have longer periods when they require little or no actual care. Ultimately, this means that the more adaptable the setting, the more the limited dollars available can be targeted toward providing services when and where they are most needed. Since remaining at home is for most people not only the most desirable but also the most flexible setting, it will be important not only to find ways of expanding home care services, but also to find ways of ensuring that people have a home to stay in. This can be accomplished through a variety of strategies, including counseling and casework services, financial assistance, and the development of appropriate congregate living settings.

Providing counseling and casework services to people with HIV and their families and friends, especially at an early point, has the potential for preventing the homelessness which can occur when people lose their jobs because of the illness, or when families become so overwhelmed with caring for their family member or friend who is ill that they give up entirely.

However, the effectiveness of such services is also dependent upon there being appropriate alternative resources available should they be needed. Rent subsidies, for example, can make the difference between keeping a home or becoming homeless, and are almost always likely to be considerably less expensive, over the long run, than the institutional alternative.

Also, much more needs to be done in making congregate living settings available to people with HIV. Several model projects have already been organized across the country, and this effort needs to continue. While some settings may be for people with HIV only, it is desirable for the reasons discussed earlier that congregate settings which integrate those with HIV with others also be developed.

In addition, the role which existing nursing homes and intermediate care settings can play for those with HIV is likely to vary somewhat among communities and will depend largely on what alternatives are available. What is essential is that people not be denied access to such facilities simply because they are suffering from HIV illness. However, it is equally crucial that care be taken in matching the services a home has to offer with the particular needs of the person with HIV illness.

Ultimately, the challenge that HIV presents for long-term care is to become more flexible, more innovative, and more sensitive to the individuals within its care. To the extent that long-term care is successful in meeting this challenge, everyone, not only those with AIDS, will benefit.

References

Bayer, Ronald. 1989. *Private acts, social consequences: AIDS and the politics of public health*. New York: Free Press.

Brandt, A. M. 1987. *No magic bullet: A social history of venereal disease in the United States since 1800*. Expanded ed. New York: Oxford University Press, Inc.

Caldwell, M. 1988. *The last crusade*. New York: Atheneum Publishers.

Committee on Nursing Home Regulation, Institute of Medicine. 1986. *Improving the quality of care in nursing homes*. Washington, D.C.: National Academy Press.

Griggs, J. Ed. *AIDS: Public policy dimensions*. 1986. Based on proceedings of the conference cosponsored by the United Hospital Fund of New York and the Institute for Health Policy Studies, School of Medicine, University of California, San Francisco, January 16 and 17.

Institute of Medicine, National Academy of Sciences. 1986. *Confronting AIDS: Directions for public health, healthcare, and research*. Washington, D.C.: National Academy Press.

Knickman, J.R., and E. Marcus. 1988. The impact of acquired immunodeficiency syndrome (AIDS) on cities. *In An urban agenda for the 1990s*, 51. New York: The Urban Research Center, Graduate School of Public Administration, New York University.

Mcheill, W.H. 1976. *Plaques and peoples*. Garden City, N.Y.: Anchor Press/Doubleday & Co. Inc.

CHAPTER 8

Ethical and Legal Concerns

Susan Harris

The relationship between laws and ethics can be perceived as interactive, with the law identifying actions that are required or prohibited—the "musts" of behavior—and ethics attempting to identify actions that are desirable—the "shoulds." The examination of behavior from an ethical perspective often results, over time, in the establishment of new legal standards. In addition, in times of change, when the appropriate legal standards are uncertain or unclear, the application of ethical considerations may be an important factor in either the development of new standards or the clarification of old ones. Thus, ethical considerations often become the foundation of law.

The presence of the human immunodeficiency virus (HIV) and the resulting cases of AIDS in contemporary society have created just such a situation, as little existing law has been directly applicable. Furthermore, limited scientific knowledge has resulted in widespread confusion about the virus and its effects. As a result, much of the law that has developed has been created by applying ethical and other considerations to the legal principles that are most nearly analogous.

Applicable Law

The most notable example of this phenomenon has been the way in which legal writers have almost unanimously applied the principles of the *School Board of Nassau County v. Arline*, a 1987 case involving tuberculosis, when considering HIV-related legal issues.

In this case, the Supreme Court stated that a contagious disease may be a handicap, as defined by Section 504 of the Rehabilitation Act of 1973, and identified the proper criteria for determining whether Ms. Arline was otherwise qualified (in that case, for continued employment) under the Act. The Rehabilitation Act prohibits refusal of employment or provision of services solely on the basis of a handicap. Employers and providers of services must provide reasonable accommodation for the special needs of the handicapped individual if an individual who can be so accommodated is considered to be "otherwise qualified" for employment or receipt of services.

The criteria identified by the Court were based on those proposed by the American Medical Association and included the determination, based on medical knowledge, of the nature, duration, severity of the risk, and probability of transmission. The court recommended deference to the reasonable medical judgment of public health officials and stated that the required reasonable accommodation analysis should be made in light of medical findings and recommendations.

Assuming that the *Arline* criteria would be applicable to HIV-positive individuals when considering both the employment and service provision requirements of the Rehabilitation Act, most legal writers agree that Medicare and Medicaid providers should consider both Section 504 and the *Arline* criteria when developing policies related to HIV-positive persons, including both actual and potential clients. In addition, many general and AIDS-specific state antidiscrimination laws are applicable. As a result, it appears that healthcare providers cannot refuse to provide care to, or employ, persons with AIDS or who are HIV-positive simply because of their condition. Although *Arline* was an employment case and the Rehabilitation Act provisions are applicable to both employment and service provision situations, this discussion will focus on the provision of service, with recognition that a similar analytical approach may be applied in employment situations.

Unfortunately, the existence of other state laws applicable to long-term care providers can create confusion. In several states, the question of whether HIV is included in specific patient and employee-related communicable disease laws which are applicable to long-term care providers is not yet resolved. Consequently, many providers believe that they may be prohibited from admitting or employing individuals known to be HIV-positive. The long-term care regulatory system is such that there are strong disincentives for providers to take action that they perceive as innovative. The possibility of a negative inspection survey finding would discourage all but the most bold.

Medicare and Medicaid regulations prohibit discharge of long-term care facility patients except for nonpayment of bills, medical emergency, or the welfare of the patient or other patients. Many states have similar requirements. (Provisions of the Omnibus Reconciliation Act of 1987 expanded these rights and provided for a discharge appeals process to be in place by October 1, 1989.) In addition, in recognition of their relatively limited resources compared with those of hospitals, long-term care facilities are prohibited from admitting individuals for whom they cannot provide care. These requirements indicate that long-term care facilities may consider their capacity to provide care to a given HIV-positive individual, whether an existing patient or an applicant for admission, as part of a Section 504 analysis.

In January, 1988, the Occupational Safety and Health Administration (OSHA) first gave notice to all healthcare employers that they must implement the Centers for Disease Control (CDC) recommendations for prevention of HIV transmission in healthcare settings (often referred to as the "CDC Guidelines" or "Universal Precautions") in order to protect healthcare employees from HIV (Department of Health and Human Services, Centers for Disease Control, August 21, 1987.) The original notice was superseded by an August 15, 1988 OSHA Instruction (CPL 2-2.44A) that incorporated the June 24, 1988 CDC update of the "Universal Precautions" and clarified OSHA requirements for healthcare employers. Consequently, not only will the CDC guidelines be applied as law by OSHA, but healthcare providers will be expected to follow certain internal administrative procedures to ensure that the guidelines are appropriately implemented.

Ethical Considerations

Several assumptions based on ethical principles are applicable to long-term care providers when considering HIV-related policies and procedures. Health care organizations have a responsibility to the community, as well as to individual clients. Staff members particularly at the professional level, have an ethical obligation to all individuals who need their services; they cannot ethically choose the most "desirable" individuals as those whom they wish to serve. Healthcare providers have a responsibility for providing accurate information to and maintaining credibility with employees, patients, families, and the community, and for ensuring that the policies and procedures they develop are responsible and sound. They must recognize the fact that in this situation, as in all situations in which an ethical analysis is required, they must weigh competing interests and values and may not be able to identify a course of action acceptable to all the affected parties. In many circumstances, they may also find that adherence to ethical principles involves risks they would not otherwise take.

Finally, providers must recognize the fear that has been generated by the HIV epidemic, and they must be willing to work to dispel it in order to meet their responsibilities to their clients and the community. In order to accomplish this objective as well as to meet other requirements and continue to provide care, it is important to acknowledge that the presence of HIV in the population mandates changes in behavior and attitude. It also requires recognizing that identification of all HIV-positive individuals is not possible at this time and as a result, a significant element of uncertainty is present in healthcare delivery. This means that no healthcare provider can realistically or responsibly avoid dealing with the presence and effects of the virus in our society.

OSHA's decision to mandate implementation of the CDC guidelines, which appears to impose an unreasonable burden on healthcare providers, is in reality an acknowledgment of the presence and effects of the virus. The decision resolves some apparently difficult questions by requiring providers of healthcare to act as though the blood and certain body fluids of all patients were infectious. Therefore, in most circumstances, and HIV-positive patient will not be identified just because special infection control procedures are implemented, thereby simplifying the problem of maintaining confidentiality. This policy also makes moot the issue of whether facilities can provide such care because all facilities are now required to be able to provide it.

Key Issues

There are still many unresolved problems and unanswered questions, some of which can be addressed and resolved by individual providers. Others, with broad public policy implications, cannot. Recognition of resource limitations in long-term care is one such issue. In many communities, long-term care beds are in short supply. In addition, shortages of all levels of staff exist almost everywhere. If long-term care services which traditionally have focused on the elderly are to be expanded to accommodate significant numbers of AIDS patients, development of additional resources must be part of a community-wide effort. Facilities, adequately trained staff, and financing must be developed in order to provide needed care in appropriate settings. No single segment of the healthcare community, be it volunteer support services, long-term care facilities, or public hospitals, can be expected to provide needed services to AIDS patients without these resources. Implementation of the CDC guidelines, although virtually eliminating the questions as to the development of adequate infection control procedures and the need to "label" known HIV-positive patients, has placed additional cost burdens on all providers for training staff and providing supplies. However, reimbursement rates have not increased to accommodate these costs, thus demonstrating another issue that cannot be adequately addressed by the individual provider. The costs of providing protection and education to patients and staff and of developing the additional resources to provide care to AIDS patients must be recognized and absorbed by the larger community.

Although long-term care providers must develop procedures which assume that any patient might be HIV-positive, they can and should also determine their ability to provide care for diagnosed AIDS patients. This is particularly true when determining whether care can be provided to a particular patient. If the individual patient's needs and the facility's ability to meet them are assessed objectively, the resulting decision should be both legally and ethically sustainable. For example, one facility may be able to care for a stable patient who requires admission primarily because of a lack of community-based services, but it may not be able to care for an acutely ill or dying patient. Another facility may be able to provide hospice-type care for the dying patient, but may not have sufficient staff expertise to provide care for a patient requiring complex drug treatments. Furthermore, few long-term care facilities have the capacity to provide care to active drug addicts. Both facility-based and home care providers may have to refuse their admission because of a lack of sufficient staff, since that additional patient would seriously compromise their ability to provide care to existing patients.

The question of whether special in-patient units for AIDS patients are necessary or desirable has thus far been considered primarily by acute care facilities. Some providers believe that such units are not only more cost effective but can better meet both the physical and psychological needs of patients. Others argue that these units are not beneficial because of the negative effects of segregation on patients and because of more rapid staff burnout. It appears that specialized units are both legally and ethically permissible if special services are actually provided and if the separation of such patients does not result in a failure to provide needed care.

Because of the size and home-like nature of long-term care facilities as well as the fact that the typical AIDS patient is noticeably different from most other long-term care facility patients, existing patients will soon realize that an AIDS patient has been admitted. Therefore, facilities will find it most appropriate to provide education to existing patients and their families, if possible, before a known AIDS patient is admitted. These psychological support and educational needs are another example of additional costs for which providers should be reimbursed as part of the societal cost of HIV.

The facility's general responsibility to the AIDS patient is no different in kind from its basic responsibility to all patients. However, the nature of the disease and the frequent negative attitudes toward persons with AIDS increase the significance of these responsibilities. Protection of confidentiality, maintenance of respect for the individual, provision of a caring and supportive environment, and attention to both physical and psychological needs may very well require additional effort when providing care to an AIDS patient.

The reactions of family members upon learning that a loved one has AIDS often require intensive staff support and/or intervention. In addition, the question of the role of the lover or special friend of an AIDS patient often raises ethical problems, especially if family members refuse to recognize either the individual or the relationship. This situation can be particularly problematic when the family tries to prevent the friend from visiting the patient or when "end of life" decisions must be made and no clear directions have been expressed by the patient. The friend or lover may often have the best knowledge of the patient's wishes but be precluded by the family from participating in the decision-making process. The facility must then struggle with the problem of how it can meet its primary responsibility to the patient within a legal framework that recognizes only traditional family relationships.

It is important to note that meeting the intensified needs of AIDS patients, providing support to their families, lovers, and friends, and resolving the problems that may arise will require significant staff time, for which either additional resources must be provided or services to other patients reduced.

Other Issues

Other legal-ethical questions which concern long-term care providers are common to the entire healthcare community, including policies and procedures for situations in which a staff member contracts AIDS or is known to be HIV-positive or in which an incident occurs such as a needlestick so that a staff member is potentially exposed to the virus. Furthermore, questions as to when or whether screening of patients and staff for HIV is appropriate, useful, or permitted are often asked. Resources from the CDC (1987a), the American Hospital Association (1987), the American Healthcare Association (1987), the American Medical Association (1987), as well as many other organizations are available to help provide answers to these questions. As with many other aspects of the impact of HIV, the primary problem is that of overcoming irrational fear. Once that has been accomplished, answers to these questions in the long-term care setting become relatively easy. There is general agreement that the risk of transmission of HIV to staff members is negligible; that screening is not useful in most circumstances; and that specific procedures should be followed when potential exposure occurs.

Conclusions

The legal-ethical issues related to long-term care and AIDS must be addressed at both the public policy and individual provider levels. Public officials have the responsibility of identifying public needs, determining priorities, and establishing mechanisms to achieve their desired objectives. They alone can make broad decisions about resource provision and allocation and clarify unclear and apparently conflicting requirements. Resources needed include not only sufficient funds to pay for care, but also for community-wide planning for and development of enough facilities and services as well as educational programs and materials suitable for varying target populations, i.e., healthcare facility staff members and the general population.

Individual providers have the responsibility to recognize and assume their roles as members of the healthcare delivery community, which may include participation in community-wide planning and decision-making processes, provision of necessary education to staff and others, and development of policies so that the facility's decision to admit the individual AIDS patient is based on an objective assessment of the facility's ability to meet that person's needs.

Finally, at both the public policy and individual provider level, a major need is the commitment of work toward overcoming irrationality and fear, so that both legal and ethical issues can be examined and resolved in a responsible and humane manner.

References

AIDS Committee. 1987. *AIDS and the nursing home.* Washington, D.C.: American Healthcare Association.

Centers for Disease Control. 1987a. Public Health Service guidelines for counseling and antibody testing to prevent HIV infection and AIDS. *Morbidity and Mortality Weekly Report* 36: 509–515.

Centers for Disease Control. 1987b. Recommendations for prevention of HIV transmission in healthcare settings. *Morbidity and Mortality Weekly Report* 36 (Supplement): 2S–18S.

Centers for Disease Control (CDC) *Recommendations for Prevention of HIV Transmission in Healthcare Settings,* Dept. of Health and Human Services, Centers for Disease Control, Aug. 21, 1987.

Council on Ethical and Judicial Affairs. 1987. *Ethical issues involved in the growing AIDS crisis.* Chicago: American Medical Association.

Department of Labor/Department of Health and Human Services. 1987. HVB/HIV. *Federal Register* 52: 41818–41824. Washington, D.C.: Government Printing Office.

OSHA Instruction CPL 2-2.44A. Aug. 15, 1988. Office of Health Compliance Assistance, U.S. Department of Labor.

Task Group on AIDS. 1987. *AIDS and the law: Responding to the special concerns of hospitals.* Chicago: American Hospital Association.

PART III

Financing
AIDS Services

CHAPTER 9

National Issues

Mary Ann Baily

Other chapters in this book discuss the unusual complexity of the needs of a person infected by the human immunodeficiency virus (HIV). Over the course of the illness, a patient may require help from the full spectrum of providers of acute medical care, mental healthcare, and personal and social services.

The financing of this care constitutes a major new burden on a healthcare system in which rising expenditures are already a serious issue. Of special concern is the financing of the heterogeneous mix of long-term care services.

The Broader Context

The issues raised by the financing of HIV-related long-term care are not new. In a financing system with many weak spots, the revenue for long-term care has traditionally been the weakest. People with extended illnesses or long-term disabilities have always had a problem paying for the care they need because it is expensive, their health status interferes with their ability to earn income and pay out of their own pockets, and third party coverage for long-term care is very limited. In 1987, for example, of the 40.6 billion dollars spent on nursing home care, 20.0 billion was paid directly by consumers and only 0.4 billion by private insurance. Most of the remainder was paid by Medicaid, which is available only to those who are impoverished (Levit and Freeland 1988).

Private insurance and Medicare have traditionally emphasized the coverage of acute medical care, especially that which is hospital-based. To the extent that the kinds of services grouped under the long-term care label were covered at all, reimbursement was structured to serve as short-term care for extended recovery from an acute episode of illness. Medicaid started with the same orientation and fell into its role as major payor for nursing home care almost accidentally. People in the categories covered by the program desperately needed the care, the cost was so high that they exhausted their resources paying for it, and there was no one else to pay.

After years of neglect, long-term care financing issues have finally caught the public's attention largely because of the increasing proportion of the population that is over 65 and therefore in the years in which the need for such care increases substantially. Major studies on the financing of long-term care for the elderly have been undertaken, and proposals for major changes have been made (Wiener, et al. 1987; Davis and Rowland 1986). Recent legislative proposals by Senators Kennedy and Mitchell and Congressman Pepper have proposed new federal roles in funding long-term care services. So far, however, these proposals have not been implemented, and the prospects for radical change in the structure of the long-term care financing system do not appear to be great.

Meanwhile, some evolutionary change has occurred in private and public third party coverage. Hospice and home healthcare benefits have been added to Medicare. State Medicaid programs are experimenting with home and community-based alternatives to nursing home care and with case management (Anderson and Fox 1987; Rowe and Ryan 1987).

In private insurance for the working age population, there has been a trend toward increased coverage of home care, hospice care, short-term nursing home care, and case management. For example, between 1984 and 1986, the percent of employees in medium and large firms with hospice benefits rose from 10 to 31% (Bureau of Labor Statistics 1987). From 1982 to 1986, the percent of employees with coverage of home healthcare increased from 32 to 66% (Short 1987).

Some improvement has occurred in catastrophic protection for the privately insured through the spread of major medical coverage with caps on total out-of-pocket expenditures on covered services and increased enrollment in health maintenance organizations (HMOs) (Short 1987). While such insurance may not include long-term care services, it improves a patient's ability to pay for them by limiting expenditures on acute care.

Coverage is less generous in smaller firms, and of course many employees have no health insurance at all (Congressional Research Service 1985). Perhaps more important, the catch-22 of employment-based health insurance for a functionally disabling illness is the effect such an illness has on the ability to work. New regulations (the Consolidated Omnibus Budget Reconciliation Act of 1986) guarantee most employees the opportunity to continue health insurance benefits at no more than 102% of group premium rates for 18 months after they become unemployed. They must, however, be able to afford the cost which is not an easy matter when income has fallen and the employer's premium contribution must now be paid by the individual.

There has been some increase in the availability of real long-term care private insurance products (policies specifically designed to pay for extended periods of care for the functionally disabled). However, the policies emphasize nursing home care, are expensive, and are targeted toward the elderly (Wiener, Ehrenworth, and Spence 1987).

Eligibility for Medicare on disability grounds takes effect only after a 29-month waiting period (five months for eligibility for disability income; two years more for Medicare). The waiting period for Medicaid eligibility is shorter (a few months); however, the applicant must be impoverished in order to qualify.

Thus, the overall financing picture for the kinds of care needed by a functionally disabled person is one of a patchwork of financing sources with much of the burden borne directly by the patient and family. The picture has improved somewhat for those who need care for a relatively short time, but it still looks very bleak for a person whose period of disability extends over a period of years. Those who need mental healthcare and personal service care have particular difficulty, since financing for these categories of service is especially limited.

Underlying Value Questions

Most Americans accept the principle that all people should have access to some level of healthcare whether or not they can afford it. In the words of the President's Commission for the Study of Ethical Problems in Medicine and Biomedical and Behavioral Research (1983), it is called an "adequate level of care." Most also believe that people who are sick should not have to forego everything else that is important to them in order to pay for healthcare; people with large medical bills should be helped.

The AIDS crisis provides compelling confirmation of this. Despite the social stigma associated with the groups at highest risk for HIV infection—homosexual males and intravenous drug abusers—and the deep fear of contagion, there seems to be agreement that victims of the disease should not simply be left to die without care.

The problem is that although there is a consensus that those who need healthcare should receive help, there is none on how much care they should get, how much of the cost they should bear themselves, and how the rest of the cost should be shared. If developing such a consensus is difficult for acute care, it is nearly impossible for long-term care. How much personal service care or mental healthcare is enough? How much responsibility do people have to provide in advance for old age or chronic disability? How much responsibility do family members have to care for each other?

Without a consensus on these important questions, healthcare financing issues are repeatedly handled on an ad hoc crisis response basis. More basic change is impossible because we are unclear about what an equitable financing system would look like.

Current Financing Patterns

The consensus on the proper division of responsibility for a person with AIDS is no clearer than it is for a 60-year-old with Alzheimer's disease or a 5-year-old with birth defects. So far, the financing of HIV-related long-term care is being handled in the usual ad hoc fashion.

Sources of financing for HIV-related care other than the patient's own resources include private insurance, Medicaid, Medicare, private charity, and public funding. The first three of these are the basic sources, but given the limits on whom they cover, what they cover, and how much they pay especially for long-term care services, they do not begin to meet the need.

Major supplementary private sources include private AIDS service organizations and foundations (often supported by volunteer effort) and uncompensated care in private hospitals. Major public sources include state and local funding of care for the indigent in general or for special HIV-related programs, and the Veterans Administration healthcare system at the federal level.

A single patient's care from infection to death may be financed by all of these sources in a complex pattern. A patient may, for example, start on a combination of private health insurance and out-of-pocket payment for uncovered services or copayments. The patient then becomes ill, loses or exhausts health insurance benefits (probably as a result of unemployment and an inability to afford premiums) and becomes eligible for Medicaid on the grounds of disability, low income, and exhaustion of assets. The patient may then manage to live long enough to qualify for Medicare while retaining eligibility for Medicaid payment of costs not covered by Medicare (which has deductibles, copayments, and premiums). Along the way, the patient may pay out-of-pocket or receive public or private charity (in the form of uncompensated care in a hospital or volunteer help at home) for services not covered by third party payment.

For private insurance and Medicaid—the most important sources of payment—financing availability varies greatly across the spectrum of patients. (Medicare is more uniform but because of the age distribution of cases and the disability waiting period, it currently plays a very small financing role.) Private insurance is provided by a multiplicity of companies, and there is great variation among policies in coverage, reimbursement, and premium structure. Medicaid is not one program but 50 individual state programs, with major variations in eligibility, services covered, and reimbursement. Moreover, some states have special programs for HIV-infected individuals within the Medicaid program which may vary in different parts of the same state.

Case management is valuable in developing a package of services to fit an individual AIDS patient's needs. Financial case management may be even more important because without help the patient may never find his way through the financing maze so that a humane, cost-effective standard of care can be identified, obtained, and paid for.

So far, not enough is known about the care HIV patients are actually receiving and the relative roles played by these different financing sources. There is a widely-held opinion that quality and economy are both served by reliance on home and community-based rather than inpatient care (for example, see the testimony before the Presidential Commission on the Human Immunodeficiency Virus Epidemic by representatives of the Blue Cross/Blue Shield Association and the Health Insurance Association of America). Nevertheless, what information exists is primarily on inpatient and outpatient hospital-based care rather than on long-term care services and is usually based on studies of the patient population served by a given institutional provider over a given time period. No studies have attempted to track all care, including long-term services provided by family, friends, and volunteers, from initial symptoms to death.

A number of research and demonstration projects now under way will soon provide better information about treatment patterns, cost, and financing. As of June, 1988, the Robert Wood Johnson Foundation had funded an AIDS health services program of demonstration projects providing comprehensive home and community-based care to AIDS patients at 9 sites selected from the 21 metropolitan areas with the largest number of AIDS patients. The Health Resources and Services Administration had funded an AIDS service delivery demonstration program with 13 projects in locations including New York City, San Francisco, Miami, and Los Angeles (Presidential Commission on the Human Immunodeficiency Virus Epidemic 1988). Anne Scitovsky of the Palo Alto Medical Foundation and James Knickman of New York University have received funding from The National Center for Health Services Research to develop cost study protocols which will then be put out to researchers to carry out. AIDS Project Lost Angeles, a home and community-based care demonstration, has generated some data on its patient population (Little et al. 1988). Private and public insurers are working on methodologies for tracking expenditures from claims data. These efforts will be aided by the recent introduction of new diagnostic codes for HIV-related disease, which will make it easier to identify HIV-related claims.

Of special interest are the few studies that follow individual patients over time. For example, Anne Scitovsky and Mary Cline, of the Palo Alto Medical Foundation and Anthony Pascal of RAND are doing several prospective cost studies that follow AIDS patients, looking at a broader range of treatment costs rather than just hospital care. Although these studies are small and geographically specific, they should provide valuable information about financing at the individual patient level.

A full-scale prospective study of a large representative sample of patients from the development of symptoms until death would, of course, be the ideal. It would, however, be very expensive and might be out of date upon completion, given the rapid rate of change in medical knowledge of HIV infection and its treatment.

Even without quantitative data, the structure of the financing system and the testimony of those responding to the care needs of the epidemic indicate that financing long-term care for HIV patients is one of the most difficult aspects of this extraordinary situation.

Critical Issues for the Future

The problems HIV patients encounter in financing long-term care are encountered by people with other conditions such as mental illness, spinal injuries, hepatitis, brain damage, terminal cancer, and Alzheimer's disease. (Where HIV patients are most unusual, perhaps, is that they face so many of the problems at once.) However, it is worthwhile to highlight features of the HIV epidemic that will be especially important for future long-term care policy.

Length of Survival

Currently, most HIV patients do not live very long after serious disability sets in. Thus, they need the types of care considered to be long-term care, but on average they do not need them for a very long time. This may change in the future.

As clinical experience accumulates, marginal improvement advances—especially treatment with antiviral drugs—can also be expected to extend life. The critical issue is the relationship between longer life expectancy and functional ability. Will patients who live longer be able to remain at work longer, or if not, will they at least be able to care for themselves? Employment status affects ability to pay for care either individually or with employment-based coverage, and functional status determines how much care is needed.

Of particular concern is the recent evidence of early cognitive changes in HIV-positive persons and the syndrome of HIV-related dementia. Experience with patients suffering from other forms of dementia such as Alzheimer's disease shows the heavy demands dementia patients can impose on the caregiving system. Cognitive loss also raises the specter of earlier loss of employment because the infected person truly cannot handle the demands of the job or because the possibility of cognitive deficits is used as an excuse for job discrimination.

If patients live longer in a state of serious disability, the issue of nursing home placement and financing will become more important. To date, HIV patients have used very little nursing home care. Nursing homes are designed for the elderly and thus are not very attractive to the predominantly young AIDS population. Moreover, nursing homes have resisted admitting AIDS patients because of high occupancy rates, low reimbursement rates in relation to their special needs, and the stigma attached to the disease. Several states have begun efforts to increase nursing home access (Rowe and Ryan, 1987). If the incidence of severe long-term HIV disability rises, such efforts will have to increase, and state Medicaid programs will have to find the funds to pay for more nursing home care.

Availability of Informal Care

The bulk of long-term care for elderly and disabled noninstitutionalized persons is traditionally provided by family and friends. However, members of the groups at highest risk of HIV infection—homosexuals and intravenous drug abusers—often lack this kind of family support. On the other hand, an inspiring network of volunteers has developed in the cities hardest hit by the epidemic. Without the thousands of hours donated by volunteers, especially members of the gay communities, the cost of care and the suffering of patients would be much greater. Nevertheless, there is a real concern about the capacity to sustain and extend this level of support as the epidemic proceeds.

Availability of Housing

The type and amount of long-term care needed by a functionally disabled person are greatly influenced by his or her living situation. For many HIV patients, especially intravenous drug abusers, the lack of suitable housing stands in the way of implementing a home and community-based treatment plan. The most dramatic example is in pediatric AIDS—the "boarder babies" who stay in the hospital at enormous cost to the Medicaid program because their mothers are HIV-infected and incapable of caring for them, and other out-of-hospital placements are not available. The housing issue is complicated by the dramatic fluctuations in need for care that characterize AIDS. A patient may require a high level of acute care to treat an episodic illness or skilled nursing to manage difficult symptoms, but between episodes may stabilize and require relatively little care. Current licensing and reimbursement policies make it difficult to offer the spectrum of care needed in a single facility, yet moving patients from one place to another is complex and difficult for the patient.

Development of appropriate residential facilities is now a priority in high incidence states such as New York, New Jersey, and California. Prototype housing arrangements have been developed and proven successful but currently must rely on ad hoc temporary funding. More stable sources of funding are needed. In cities that already could not cope with increasing numbers of homeless people, however, finding the resources to house this new group will be very difficult.

Extra Costs

HIV patients may need more units of care, i.e., more frequent home care visits, more extensive counseling services, and additional supplies, than other long-term care patients. Moreover, each unit of care may cost more to provide.

Special infection control precautions raise costs. These precautions require additional nursing time, use additional supplies, and increase training costs because staff members must be taught the procedures. For both medical and psychosocial reasons, management of the HIV patient is more complex than management of the average long-term care patient, and therefore increases nursing requirements. Finally, the emotional strains of dealing with the deaths of young terminally ill patients day after day as well as the fears of contagion are likely to lead to staff exhaustion and burnout. To counteract this, providers may need to invest in supportive mental health services for them.

Such extra costs are important for an assessment of the magnitude of the financing burden. They are also important for assessment of the adequacy of third party reimbursement. If payment systems do not reflect these costs, access to care is likely to suffer, and the financial problems of uncompensated care will be created for the providers who do accept HIV patients. Current reimbursement systems generally do not incorporate extra HIV-related costs, although some states are experimenting with special rates, and the Presidential Commission has recommended the federal Medicaid regulations allow supplemental reimbursement for services to HIV patients.

Specialization in the Care of HIV Patients

Whether HIV patients should be isolated in separate facilities or cared for by providers who specialize in HIV-related care is not only a quality of care issue, but also one of cost and financing. Is specialized care cost effective and if so, how should it be reimbursed?

Stigma Associated with the Disease

Even if any extra resource costs associated with caring for these patients are fully reimbursed, providers may avoid them because of their own negative attitudes toward the disease or their fear that taking HIV patients will spoil their ability to attract other types of patients. Additional reimbursement for AIDS patient care may be necessary to overcome this reluctance and to ensure a sufficient supply of services. This is particularly important in an environment in which the availability of long-term care services is being rationed as a matter of public policy, as for example, in states restricting the number of nursing home beds.

Response of Private Insurers

Currently, private insurance is not a major payor for long-term care services. However, if people at risk for HIV infection are excluded from standard health insurance or must pay much higher premiums for it, their out-of-pocket costs for the acute care costs of the illness will be greater, they will use up their financial resources more rapidly, and they will become dependent on public programs more quickly.

So far, most insurers (or self-insured employers) consider HIV-related disease just another serious illness and handle it as well or as badly as they do cancer, diabetes, or heart disease. Employees who have employment-related group insurance are generally covered without reference to individual risk factors. Those who try to obtain their insurance on an individually underwritten basis because they work for small firms or are not offered employment-related insurance have difficulty obtaining insurance if their health histories indicate an elevated risk of HIV or other disease.

There is reason for concern, however, that as insurers and employers increase their ability to monitor expenditures on HIV infection they will look for ways to limit their exposure, especially if expenditures increase significantly over current levels. This could involve excluding HIV-related costs from coverage or screening employees for elevated risk of disease.

On the other hand, the very real savings that can result from keeping AIDS patients out of the hospital may accelerate existing trends toward coverage of a broader range of out-of-hospital services provided in a case management context for all patients.

Conclusions

HIV infection puts new strains on a long-term care financing system already in crisis. The questions raised are familiar. How can the resources available to those in need of long-term care be efficiently increased by insurance or other mechanisms? How can third party coverage be structured to encourage the provision of cost-effective services tailored to the individual patient's situation, given the great variation in needs among patients and over time? How can coordination be achieved between the formal and informal, the public and private, the medical and nonmedical sectors, so they are complements rather than substitutes? How can all this be done in the absence of a philosophical framework to guide decisions, since it is unlikely that there will be one developed in the near future?

In addition, the special attention the HIV epidemic is receiving raises a question of equity. How can the needs of this group of patients be met without unfairness to others whose needs are also great? In a time of constrained healthcare resources, measuring the needs of one group against another is a painful task. The addition of a whole new group of people to the competition for scarce resources makes the task even more painful. HIV patients are no less deserving than other patients, but they are no more deserving either. Ideally, this new crisis will be met with reforms in long-term care financing that will benefit all those who need it rather than only those who have been infected by HIV.

References

Anderson, M.D. and P.D. Fox. 1987. Lessons learned from Medicaid managed care approaches. *Health Affairs* 6: 71–86.

Bureau of Labor Statistics. 1987. *Employee benefits in medium and large firms, 1986.* Washington, D.C.: Government Printing Office.

Congressional Research Service. 1988. *Health insurance and the uninsured: Background data and analysis.* Prepared for the Committees on Education and Labor and Energy and Commerce, U.S. House of Representatives, and Special Committee on Aging, U.S. Senate. Washington, D.C.: Government Printing Office.

Davis, K., and D. Rowland. 1986. *Medicare policy: New directions for health and long-term care.* Baltimore: Johns Hopkins University Press.

Rowe, M. and C. Ryan. 1987. *AIDS: A public health challenge. Vol. 2: Managing and financing the problem.* Developed for the Public Health Service of the U.S. Department of Health and Human Services under Contract 282-05-0013. Washington, D.C.: Intergovernmental Health Policy Project.

Levit, K.R., and M.S. Freeland. 1988. Data watch: National medical care spending. *Health Affairs* 7: 124–136.

Little, J., et al. 1988. AIDS home health, attendant or hospice care: Pilot study—April 1, 1986 to May 31, 1987. Los Angeles: AIDS Project Los Angeles.

Presidential Commission for the Study of Ethical Problems in Medicine and Biomedical and Behavioral Research. 1983. *Securing access to healthcare.* Vol. 1. Washington, D.C.: Government Printing Office.

Presidential Commission on the Human Immunodeficiency Virus Epidemic. 1988. *Report of the Presidential Commission on the Human Immunodeficiency Virus Epidemic.* Washington, D.C.: Government Printing Office.

Short, P.F. 1988. Trends in employee health insurance benefits. *Health Affairs* 7: 186–196.

Wiener, J.M., D.A. Ehrenworth, and D.A. Spence. 1987. Private long-term care insurance: Cost, coverage and restrictions. *The Gerontologist* 27: 487–493.

Wiener, J.M. et al. 1987. Financing and organizational options for long-term care. Testimony presented at a hearing on long-term care, Subcommittee on Health, Ways and Means Committee, U.S. House of Representatives, March 31, 1987.

CHAPTER 10

Focus on State Roles in Financing Options

Richard E. Merritt

It is unrealistic to expect a massive infusion of new federal dollars to finance the health and long-term care service needs of AIDS patients. Hence, it is important to think about what can be done within the confines of the existing fragmented healthcare financing system. The problem of financing services for AIDS patients must be viewed within the broader context of the social problem that currently exists—financing healthcare services for the medically indigent and uninsured. Those with AIDS, AIDS-related conditions, or those who are asymptomatic but antibody-positive are a growing subgroup of the broad uninsured population.

The Current State Financing System

The United States healthcare financing system has been described as having three dimensions:

1. it is a fringe benefit for most of the employed;
2. it is an entitlement conditioned by categorical eligibility for many, e.g., Medicaid and Medicare; and
3. it is a matter of chance and charity for all the rest.

The question is, what are state governments doing, or what can they do, to reduce the overall reliance by those who are indigent and uninsured on chance and charity?

Considerable attention has been devoted to the cost of providing medical care for AIDS patients. The costs per case have been coming down primarily because more emphasis is being placed on outpatient services and case management and less on hospitalization (Hellinger 1988). That is the good news. The bad news, particularly from the states' point of view, is that there is growing evidence that the costs of financing care for AIDS patients are shifting away from the private sector and more and more toward the public sector, particularly the state and local governments. Such evidence includes the following:

1. The federal government still requires a two-year waiting period for disability benefits under Medicare in addition to the five month waiting period for disability eligibility.

2. We also know that private insurers are restricting eligibility by using AIDS antibody testing or other screening mechanisms.

3. Employer efforts to curtail healthcare costs have reduced traditional cross-subsidies of providing care for the poor.

States have two broad options for addressing the inadequacy of health insurance coverage of those with human immunodeficiency virus (HIV) infection. They can adopt policies designed to enhance private health insurance coverage for AIDS patients and they can expand coverage for AIDS patients under a publicly financed program.

It is important to understand that individuals with AIDS or AIDS-related conditions have a greater likelihood of not having health insurance coverage for several reasons:

1. People who are self-employed or who work in small businesses are less likely to have private health insurance coverage, and gay men (who comprise the majority of AIDS cases) are disproportionately represented among the self-employed.

2. Losing a job because of an illness often means the loss of health insurance.

3. In many states, health and life insurance companies are requiring applicants for individual health policies in excess of certain thresholds to take a test for the presence of HIV antibodies. This contributes to an increased number of uninsured as those who test positive for the virus and are excluded from coverage. Many others never even apply because they are afraid of the consequences of discrimination.

Options for States

What options do states have for addressing these problems? First, they can restrict the conditions under which the AIDS antibody test can be used for determining insurability. However, major arguments have already arisen between the health and life insurance industry on the one hand, and associations representing gay rights and persons with AIDS over this issue. The insurance industry, however, argues that in order to write an individual health insurance policy, companies must have access to all medically relevant information about the individual applicant, including whether or not he or she is positive for antibodies to HIV. Opponents argue that the antibody test itself really does not prove who will actually contract AIDS. It merely identifies those who are antibody-positive and therefore is not a good test for actuarial purposes. Insurers counter by saying that the business of insurance is based not upon certainties but upon probabilities of outcome, and in that regard, submit that a person who is seropositive has a mortality rate 26 times greater than one of the same age cohort who is seronegative.

A few states have adopted legislation or regulations to restrict the conditions under which insurance companies can apply the antibody test for determining insurability. The District of Columbia is clearly the most restrictive in this area. Approved in 1986, the District's law prohibits insurers from using any test for identifying exposure to HIV to determine eligibility for coverage or for setting rates for five years. As a result of the law, however, many insurance companies have ceased writing individual policies in the District. As a spokesman for the health insurance industry points out,

Arbitrarily setting limits on the use of medical information allows people infected with HIV to obtain insurance at a price that does not truly reflect the risk they represent, resulting in an indirect subsidy by lower risk policyholders (Schramm 1988).

A second approach is to ensure that alternative insurance coverage or financial assistance is available to those excluded from private health insurance. States can choose from a number of options to effect this goal.

One option, so far adopted by 15 states, is to create a so-called health insurance risk pool. Many of these risk pools have been around since the mid-1970s, long before the HIV was discovered. Nevertheless, the AIDS epidemic has generated renewed interest in this financing option. Basically, a risk pool is created by a law mandating the participation of all insurance companies in an association authorized to sell health insurance within a state's boundaries. These associations, or pools, offer a comprehensive health insurance plan to individuals who, because of pre-existing conditions, are deemed uninsurable and cannot otherwise obtain private health insurance coverage. These plans are characterized by very high deductibles and co-insurance. Premiums are also very high, and usually they are insufficient to cover the losses of the plan. These losses are therefore covered by assessing each of the participating companies in proportion to their share of the state insurance market.

A primary stumbling block to the risk pool option as a major financing strategy is that federal law prohibits states from regulating self-insured plans. Hence, companies that self-insure cannot be required to participate and share the financial risk in the various state risk pool programs. The result is that Blue Cross and the commercial health insurance companies must bear a greater share of the financial risk. The state of Maine found a way around this hurdle by financing its risk pool largely through a tax on hospitals' operating revenues. Illinois supports its program through general revenues. The only other way around this obstacle would be for the federal government to permit states to regulate self-insured plans and thus include them in the base to share in the financial losses of the pool.

Other strategies that states have used to expand private health insurance coverage opportunities have included

1. prohibiting insurance underwriting practices from using information on sexual orientation;

2. mandating that employers allow employees to continue their group health insurance policy for several months following their termination from the job or to convert their coverage to individual policies; and

3. insisting that certain benefits, e.g., mental health, hospice, and home healthcare, be offered as part of group health insurance plans.

In addition, a few states have authorized tax credits or deductions for individuals willing to provide for a disabled relative or friend in their home.

A variety of other approaches have been introduced in a few states that, if enacted, would also lead to expanded health insurance coverage for persons with AIDS. For example, a bill in the Oregon Senate advocates taxing cigarettes an extra three cents a pack and directing the funds toward offsetting the costs of long-term care services for AIDS patients. A Pennsylvania House bill would appropriate $20 million to provide back-up financial assistance for healthcare services for AIDS patients after all other funding mechanisms are exhausted.

The Role of Medicaid

The largest source of public funds for the support of AIDS patients is the joint federal-state Medicaid program. An estimated 40% of all AIDS patients have at least part of their care financed by Medicaid, and about 23% of the healthcare costs of AIDS patients nationally are paid by Medicaid. During fiscal year 1987, the Healthcare Financing Administration estimated that about $400 million in Medicaid funds was spent on medical services for people with AIDS. That figure is expected to reach $600 million in fiscal year 1988. Nevertheless, because states have broad latitude in determining both who may qualify for Medicaid services and the extent of the benefit package, considerable variation exists with respect to coverage. Andrulis's recent analysis (1987) concluded that approximately 60% of persons with AIDS in the Northeast qualified for Medicaid compared with only 15% in the South.

Medicaid is not a financing system to cover a specific disease; rather it is a system to provide services for individuals who are eligible by virtue of certain categorical circumstances, e.g., low income mothers with dependent children, or low income aged, blind, or disabled persons. While all individuals with a confirmed diagnosis of AIDS are automatically presumed to be disabled according to a Social Security Administration ruling, only those whose income and resources qualify them for financial assistance under the Supplemental Security Income program generally qualify for Medicaid benefits as well.

There are a number of things states can do and are doing within the context of their Medicaid programs that target benefits to the needs of persons with AIDS.

To begin, 47 of the 50 states have agreed to cover the cost of the azidothymidine (AZT) drug for persons with AIDS who qualify for Medicaid. AZT is the only antiviral drug so far approved by the FDA, and to date it has demonstrated promising results in decreasing the severity of episodic infections and lengthening the survival time of those who take it. Without such coverage, the drug's annual cost of $8,000 or more would make it inaccessible to thousands of AIDS patients.

Many states have reported that Medicaid-eligible persons with AIDS (PWAs) have difficulty gaining access to some services already covered by Medicaid. The most frequently reported problem is access to nursing home beds. The problem is complicated by the fact that most skilled and intermediate care facilities are already operating at close to full occupancy. However, other considerations such as the heavy care needs of many PWAs, the low Medicaid reimbursement rates, and the fear of patient and family reactions, all add up to making nursing home services the major gap in the continuum of care needs of PWAs.

This situation has tremendous cost implications since on the one hand, better management of the AIDS disease means that many patients survive longer and require less hospitalization. On the other hand, many of those individuals are still maintained in expensive hospital beds beyond appropriate times simply because no post-acute care beds are available.

What are states doing to address this problem? Recently, the Illinois legislature authorized "quality incentive payments" to nursing homes to accommodate the special needs of patients with AIDS or AIDS-related complex (ARC) (Public Act 85-684, 1987 Laws). Wisconsin has received federal approval for special reimbursement rates for the development of subacute care units in hospitals to treat AIDS patients. A few states are considering an expedited review process under their certificate of need programs for applications for projects to construct or modify facilities for the care and treatment of PWAs.

The state of Minnesota confronted head on the issue of discrimination against AIDS patients by nursing homes. The state's Department of Human Rights sued 17 nursing homes that had denied access to AIDS patients. A settlement was reached whereby the nursing homes agreed to assess persons with AIDS based on their need for medical care rather than on their diagnostic status. Also, the nursing homes have agreed to provide training to staff members to work with AIDS patients.

> The actions by the Human Rights Department have established that AIDS is not a condition which nursing homes may use as a basis for denying access to care, and that the Human Rights Department will demand that healthcare professionals and the community provide services to AIDS patients (Minnesota Department of Health 1988, 54).

While a skilled nursing or intermediate care facility may be the most appropriate setting for some AIDS patients, clearly the preferred choice of most following discharge from a hospital is some form of home or community-based care. A key provision (Section 2176) of the Omnibus Budget Reconciliation Act of 1981 gave life to this option. Until that time, Medicaid policy was extraordinarily biased toward institutional long-term care. However, with the advent of the Section 2176 provision, the federal government agreed to provide Medicaid payments to states for certain non-Medicaid services believed to be effective in reducing or eliminating the need for more costly institutional care. Such services might include respite care, for example, or adult day care.

States, however, were obliged to obtain a waiver of federal Medicaid rules from the Secretary of the Department of Health and Human Services in order to implement such a program. The waivers were contingent in part on the state's ability to show that the services it proposed to offer were more cost effective than the services now being provided.

As originally intended, states that were successful in obtaining a waiver for home and community-based services could target the services to the needs of specific population groups, i.e., the elderly or disabled, but not to a specific diagnosis. In 1986, however, Congress modified the law to allow states to establish a diagnosis of AIDS as a criterion for recipient access to waivered services.

Currently, only four states (New Jersey, New Mexico, Ohio, and Hawaii) have received waivers to provide home and community-based services for people with AIDS. However, at least two other states have applications pending, and several others are considering submitting applications.

New Jersey's three-year waiver became effective on March 1, 1987. The program is geared primarily toward addressing the needs of the state's intravenous drug-using population with AIDS or ARC as well as their infected children. Specific services offered under the waiver include individual and continuous private duty nursing care, case management, personal care assistant services, certain narcotic and drug abuse treatments at home, and intensive supervision of children with AIDS or ARC who live in supervised foster homes.

Eligibility for these services is limited to those who have a confirmed diagnosis of AIDS or ARC and are in need of institutional care. The state estimates that the program will serve up to 350 individuals during the first year of operation, 600 in the second year, and 1,000 in the third.

New Mexico's program emphasizes a coordinated community in-home care approach for persons with AIDS or ARC. Specific services included under the waiver are homemaker and personal care services to assist the individual with daily functioning, adult day care services, and private duty nursing. Approximately 74 persons will receive service at an average estimated cost per person of $36,000 annually. The state estimates that in the absence of these alternative services, the annual cost per person would be $59,000.

Recently, Congress expanded the list of optional services that states can provide and receive matching federal payments under Medicaid. The two new services, hospice and case management, while not available exclusively for AIDS patients, should be of considerable benefit to PWAS who need them. It is well known that the medical and social service needs of the AIDS patient are diverse and complex, and a good case manager can provide an essential coordinating function in linking the client with the most appropriate array of services. Case managers can also help facilitate discharges of AIDS patients who are no longer in need of acute care services but for whom limited community-based alternatives exist. Hospice services provide a humane alternative for those AIDS patients who choose to forego medical treatment for their illness and want only palliative care.

In some states, low income individuals who cannot quality for Medicaid may be eligible for some form of state-only assistance program or state and local government assistance. These programs vary dramatically from state to state, but where they exist they can be an important source of support for indigent patients, including those with AIDS.

Indigent Care Programs

State-operated indigent care programs exist in more than two-thirds of the states. Most of these are associated with a state or county general assistance program, which usually includes a medical services components. States with a high incidence of AIDS such as California, New York, and New Jersey report that their general assistance medical programs are filling an important gap for HIV-infected persons who do not qualify for Medicaid. Services covered under the general assistance medical programs in New York and New Jersey are essentially the same as those provided to the categorically needy population under Medicaid—hospital, laboratory, physician, skilled nursing, rural health clinic, and family planning.

Since these programs do not benefit from federal funds, they also are not affected by federal regulations. Hence, states are free to tailor them to improve the range of services available to HIV-infected individuals. For example, services could be broadened to include adult day healthcare, nonemergency transportation, outpatient drug therapy, and respite care.

Programs for Target Populations

Another state-only financing strategy involves targeting resources to the needs of special populations. Florida, Maryland, and Missouri, for example, have state-funded and administered prenatal assistance programs. While these programs are designed to reduce infant mortality rates and improve birth outcomes, they are also well suited to the early diagnosis and treatment of children born to women who are intravenous drug users. Massachusetts and New Jersey have also allocated considerable state resources for medical care and social services unique to the needs of intravenous drug users.

Another possible model for financing health services for HIV-infected persons is that of a disease-specific program. Several states operate small programs for people suffering from such illnesses as renal disease, sickle cell anemia, cancer, and hemophilia. As the range of services and the number of persons serviced can be quite restrictive, this model should be viewed as a supplement to, not a substitute for, investment in a better health insurance program either under the auspices of general assistance or Medicaid. However, a disease-specific program could fill some gaps in coverage for individuals with AIDS.

In Florida, for example, a disease-specific program model is being used to provide significant benefits to individuals with AIDS. In a state such as Florida where no general assistance program exists, direct funding may be the only avenue possible until and unless the indigent care burden is addressed more comprehensively.

In fiscal 1986–1987, some $4.2 million of Florida's general revenues will go to Jackson Memorial Medical Center to develop an AIDS patient care network in Dade County. Jackson Memorial is expected to provide approximately $3 million in direct inpatient and outpatient services and to subcontract for another $2 million for essential home health, hospice, transportation, and psychosocial services. The legislature intends the Jackson Memorial AIDS network to serve as a model for other counties; to that end, it has appropriated an additional $700,000 for AIDS patient care among the five other counties with the highest incidences of AIDS. In the Florida AIDS network, the state appropriation will pay for care for noninsured AIDS individuals, certain relevant services not covered by Medicaid, and the difference between reimbursement levels under Medicaid and Medicare for any Medicaid eligibles approved for a supplementary rate increase for physician and home healthcare services.

Assuring Access

If lack of access to care (primary, tertiary, or long-term) for AIDS patients escalates into a serious problem, states may begin to force some degree of availability under their regulatory authority. For example, proposals to tie licensure or certificate of need approval to a facility's willingness to accept a certain number of AIDS patients may become more common. A few states already condition the approval of certificate of need applications to a facility's plan for serving indigent patients, and each year measures are introduced in a few state legislatures requiring physicians to treat Medicaid patients as a condition of relicensure.

Conclusion

States are on the front line of support care for AIDS patients and for funding long-term care services for all populations in need. Clearly, states have a wide range of strategies which they can, and are, using to address the financing of care. By adopting policies which influence private insurance coverage and by expanding public health benefits, state governments can have significant impact on access to care. In the last few years, several states have experimented in both of these policy frontiers. States can take a leadership role in creative program development and testing for the long-term care of AIDS patients and other appropriate populations.

References

Andrulis, D. 1987. The provision and financing of medical care for AIDS patients in U.S. public and private teaching hospitals. *Journal of the American Medical Association* 258: 1343–1346.

Hellinger, F.J. 1988. Forecasting personal medical care costs of AIDS from 1988 through 1991. *Journal of American Public Health* 103:313.

Minnesota Department of Health. 1988. *Report of the Minnesota Interagency Committee on AIDS Financing Issues* Feb.: 54.

Schramm, C.J. 1988. Insurers advocate HIV testing. AIDS *Patient Care* 2: 4–6.

PART IV

Issues of
Public Policy

CHAPTER 11

Provider Perspective:
A Double Dilemma

L. Gregory Pawlson and Lois A. Wiechmann

In some respects a consideration of public policy issues overlaps with issues addressed in the financing and delivery of long-term care for persons with AIDS and other human immunodeficiency virus (HIV) related diseases. This chapter will focus on three fundamental questions that are likely to involve significant public debate and discussion.

1. What proportion of financing for long-term care of persons with HIV-related diseases should be public and at what organizational level (i.e., local, regional, state, or federal)?

2. Should eligibility for these services be universal or means-tested?

3. Should services be usual and customary (i.e., integrated with those for other diseases) or separate (i.e., disease-specific)?

This chapter will examine these questions from the perspective of existing policy (whether explicit or implicit), provide a rationale for an optimal policy in each area, and finally consider what is most likely to occur given the dominant political and social factors in the United States.

HIV appears to have a propensity for affecting both the individual and society in very vulnerable areas. The biology of HIV is such

129

that it attaches preferentially via a receptor (termed the CD4 receptor) to the surface of cells, most often the T4 lymphocytes, involved in the body's defense against microorganisms (viruses, bacteria, fungi, etc.). After a period of latency, genetic materials from the virus which have been incorporated into the host cell, "take over" certain functions, resulting in cellular dysfunction and eventual cell death. Loss of these lymphocytes impairs the body's ability to fight most microorganisms (Fauci 1987).

Through the clinical syndromes of AIDS and other less well-defined entities, the effect of the virus on healthcare services and financing in the United States is devastating. Populations hardest hit by HIV-related diseases are subsegments of the population who are outside the political and social mainstream. In one group, intravenous drug users, the infection results from an illegal activity, and in another, homosexuals, it results from activities that are feared, denied, or derided by large segments of the population.

Additionally, HIV-related diseases are contagious (albeit in very specific circumstances which require far more than casual contact), cause significant losses in the ability to function in activities crucial to living in the community, and are nearly always fatal. Diseases with these characteristics are handled poorly in our society, with our actions being driven by fear rather than rational debate (Arno 1986; Iglehart 1987; Brandt 1988).

Adding the issues surrounding long-term care to those of HIV-related diseases results in an even more difficult and complex problem for our society. Explicit long-term care policy in the United States is almost nonexistent. Fragmentation of services, barriers to access, and inadequacy and inequity of financing are unfortunately the hallmarks of long-term care in this country. These problems are clearly compounded when the use of long-term care by populations who have HIV-related disorders is considered. A few examples illustrate the extent of the problems we face.

The burden imposed on home care, or nursing home care providers is especially heavy when both intensive, active treatment for a potentially transmissible disease and severe functional impairment are present in the same patient at the same time. The problems posed by persons with HIV-related diseases impose additional burdens. The generally low socioeconomic status of many of the victims and the high cost of care during acute exacerbations and complications of the illness expose the inadequacies of the financing of long-term care services in this country (Arno 1986). Fears of providers and of elderly long-term care residents and their families of having persons with HIV-positive diseases in long-term care settings illuminate the isolation and lack of training and education characteristic of most-long-term care settings (Marlowe 1987; Gillis 1987). Finally, the apparent changing incidence, prevalence, definition, and course of HIV-related disease make planning of long-term care even more difficult. Basic information regarding what proportion of those infected with HIV will develop which type of disease, or what effect on function and survival the use of azidothymidine (AZT) and other drugs will have on patients is still unclear (Fauci 1987; Rothenberg et al. 1987).

Current Policies and Patterns

Having identified the extent and complexity of public policy concerns surrounding long-term care of those with HIV-related diseases, we turn to an examination of current policies (or lack thereof) prior to determining what an optimal policy should be or what policies are likely to be initiated.

While efforts in biomedical research related to HIV are now, after some delay, extensive and reasonably well coordinated (via the Department of Health and Human Services, with the Centers for Disease Control and the National Institutes of Health playing prominent roles), approaches to financing or delivery of care are largely unplanned or nonexistent (Arno 1986; Iglehart 1987; New York Times Editorial 1988; Rudensky 1986; Fruen 1988; Laudicina 1987; Rowe and Ryan 1988; Buchanan 1988). The development of a rational public policy has been hampered by widespread fears about AIDS and the relatively weak political power of the populations most affected by it (with San Francisco perhaps as the exception). In addition, our tendency to blame the victim for the disease is a considerable barrier to progress. The fact that AIDS is a venereal disease also clearly influences our handling of the problem (Brandt 1988). A number of task forces and advisory panels have been formulated to address various aspects of the HIV problem, but in general, they too have tended to focus on areas other than the financing and delivery of services to those already infected (Iglehart

1987). It is more politically advantageous to talk about preventing the spread of the disease (especially to the white upper middle class) than to finance or deliver services to homosexuals or intravenous drug users with established disease. Indeed, it seems that our clearest policy toward the financing and delivery of long-term care services to those with HIV-related disorders is to avoid recognizing responsibility or taking action.

Thus, the vast majority of funding and services for the care of persons with HIV-related diseases has fallen on the patchwork of existing healthcare programs. Since most healthcare coverage for the nonelderly population is through employers, many AIDS victims, either because they are not employed or because they have become unemployed because of disability, are without insurance. State financing or service programs for the indigent have therefore assumed a major role in the crisis (Arno 1986; Sisk 1987). A few states such as New York and California have embarked on developing comprehensive care centers which include elements for both acute and chronic disease (Arno 1986; Rowe and Ryan 1988). A recent survey compiled by the Intergovernmental Health Policy Project noted that state-only funding for all AIDS-related activities varied from over $2 per capita in New York and California to $0.003 in Iowa (Rowe and Ryan 1988). While the survey also found that the relative proportion of state-only funding going to direct patient care services was growing (from 4% in 1986 to 16% in 1988), no information was given as to the distribution between acute and long-term care.

Because of financial barriers created by problems with financing, much of the care of patients with HIV-positive disease—especially long-term care—has fallen to public hospitals and those providers willing to accept the limited reimbursement available from Medicaid or from state public health programs (Rowe and Ryan 1988; Andrulis 1987). At present, it is estimated that about 25% of all financing for care provided to AIDS victims is derived from Medicaid alone (Buchanan 1988). How much of that payment goes for long-term care services is unknown. Since Medicaid supplies nearly half of the funding for all long-term care services in this country, it is likely that it is the major source of funding for AIDS victims with such needs.

The ability of AIDS victims to apply for Medicaid was improved by a Social Security Administration decision to allow the diagnosis of AIDS (but not other HIV-related diseases) to be a presumptive determination of disability. Having a disability and meeting certain asset and income criteria determine eligibility for Supplemental Security Income payments, which in turn, in many states, allows access to Medicaid. There are significant problems with Medicaid-based financing of care, including the variability of benefits from state to state, the inadequate reimbursement and subsequent limited access to providers in many states, and the statutory limits in the Medicaid program which inhibit the development of programs tailored to the needs of persons with AIDS. While state Medicaid agencies are still prohibited from altering or adding special benefits for a single disease, Congress has passed legislation that allows states to implement alternative approaches for all recipients which include expanded home-based care, case management, and hospice programs. Waivers for such programs must be reviewed and approved by specific federal agencies, e.g., the Healthcare Financing Administration. The waivers must show the cost effectiveness of the program, the effect on proposed recipients, and how it fits into the Medicaid programs (Smith 1986).

With longer survival and the presumption of disability under Social Security, more persons with AIDS may eventually receive Medicare coverage. This would occur after the two-year waiting period following the presumption of disability. Since survival for certain forms of AIDS now exceeds two years and increased survival is expected with certain drug therapies (Rothenberg et al. 1987), Medicare coverage could become much more frequent. While Medicare has no true long-term care benefits, the postacute hospital nursing home and home care benefits would be very useful for AIDS patients. To the extent that the elderly pay for Medicare benefits, they may end up contributing a disproportionate share of the expenses of those with AIDS. While in general the elderly finance less than 10% of Medicare, they will pay 100% for some benefits, including drugs in the recently enacted Medicare "catastrophic" expansion.

Because many of the early victims of AIDS were young employed homosexuals, private insurance has provided some reimbursement for the care of those with HIV-related diseases. This proportion is likely to diminish if the increase in the proportion of intravenous drug users in the HIV-positive disease population continues and longer survival and disability ensues. Although few private insurance programs cover a significant amount of long-term care, a number of programs, and especially those involving health maintenance organizations, cover posthospital home care as an effort to limit hospitalization. Legislation passed by Congress in 1985 has increased the possibility that private insurance will be available for a limited number of persons with AIDS when it required that anyone whose employment was terminated be allowed to continue their medical coverage at 102% of the employer's cost if the employer had more than 20 employees. This would allow persons with AIDS who become unemployed the opportunity to purchase private insurance for an additional 18 months. The limitations, however, are obvious. The insurance would be more expensive than the usual employee copay and would come at a time when the individual's income has been reduced or terminated. Private insurance companies are strong advocates of the use of screening new policyholders for HIV to avoid the adverse risk associated with insuring persons with AIDS (Iglehart, Read, and Wells 1987; Faden and Kass 1988). Since private insurance companies increase profitability by avoiding high risk patients— whether the risk is with AIDS, diabetes, or emphysema—it is likely that private insurance will play a limited role in underwriting care for HIV-related diseases.

In the case of homosexuals with HIV-related diseases, much of the case management and coordination (and in many cases the actual delivery of care) in some areas has been provided by volunteer organizations in the gay-lesbian community. That model may well not apply to the growing population of HIV-infected patients who are intravenous drug users (Laudicina 1987).

Services for those with HIV-related diseases are currently provided both separately and integrated with existing services. While there have been attempts to develop facilities or services specifically for those with AIDS, in general it appears that most direct care is given by providers and in facilities that care for other populations as well. Provider fears of possible transmission of HIV to other patients or to themselves have been problematic in long-term care settings and may tend to force clustering of persons with HIV-related diseases into a few facilities or programs (Arno 1986; Marlowe 1987).

There is also a recognition that some long-term care service providers lack the skills and training to provide the intensity and skill level of services often required by those with HIV-related diseases (Marlowe 1987; Gillis 1987). Another barrier is the lack of a consistent policy on the reimbursement of long-term care providers. Some states such as Florida, New York, and Wisconsin have provided special reimbursement for those nursing homes willing to treat patients with AIDS. The results of such programs are as yet uncertain (Laudicina 1987; Rowe and Ryan 1988). We are not aware of any current data which detail the use of long-term care services by those with HIV-related diseases, let alone whether such services are provided in general or disease-specific settings.

Toward an Optimal Solution

Given the uneven geographic distribution of HIV-positive diseases in the population, the disproportionate numbers of individuals with low income who are affected, and the catastrophic nature of the illness (both in terms of cost and effect on function), there would seem to be a strong argument for publicly financed insurance coverage of long-term care for individuals with AIDS. Indeed, the same argument could be made for similar coverage for all severe chronic illness. There is a reasonable rationale for encouraging (or requiring) the purchase of prefunded, private long-term care insurance, given the limited risk but high cost of long-term care (Institute of Medicine, National Academy of Sciences 1986) in the older population. However, the cost of HIV-related diseases is spread over a much smaller population, with the risk of developing the disease almost certain in a group that is easily identified—those with positive HIV titers (Fauci 1987). Thus, most of the recommendations of the task force appointed by Congress to suggest solutions to the problems of financing long-term care for the elderly are simply not applicable to the HIV-positive population (Institute of Medicine, National Academy of Sciences 1986). It appears that our only viable alternative is a program that is publicly financed.

If we would proceed to a publicly financed program, the question arises as to whether the program should be means-tested, and whether financing or services should be state or federal. First, given the unequal distribution of HIV disease, unless one believes that the general public in San Francisco or New York is largely responsible for the epidemic in their area, it is hard to imagine why we should rely heavily on state or local funding. In addition, state determination of eligibility is likely to produce the same uneven pattern of coverage as in the Medicaid program. On the basis of both efficacy and equity, it is suggested that there should be a federally financed, non-means-tested program based on revenues from general income tax or a similarly progressive tax. High cost, recurrent, and specialized services (excluding basic room and board) could then be provided with universal eligibility for those with chronic long-term care needs, regardless of the cause.

The public debate around the issue of whether to segregate long-term services for those with HIV-positive diseases will no doubt be long and heated. The risk of segregation in terms of discrimination both in access to and payment for services is considerable. For example, it might be difficult to attract and keep an adequate quality and quantity of providers in such programs. Yet, the fact that most current long-term care services are oriented to the needs and characteristics of the frail elderly is also a major consideration. Anyone who has cared for a young person in a nursing home where the average age of residents approaches 85 knows these limitations (Marlowe 1987). Furthermore, the need for relatively intensive ongoing treatment in most persons with HIV-related diseases who also require long-term care is problematic. As noted previously, providers in many home care and nursing homes are not suitably trained or equipped to handle such patients. It would seem that a combination of specialized programs, as for example, a hybrid chronic care/acute care hospital with home care and hospice services might be ideal. A key issue would be to provide reimbursement sufficient to ensure effective humane care in these settings. In communities with a lower prevalence of the disease, integration with existing community facilities would seem to be the most reasonable approach.

What Is Likely to Be

Given the polarized nature of political views toward HIV-positive diseases in the Administration and Congress, i.e., witness the acerbic debates on AIDS between Jessie Helms and Lowell Weicker that seem to occur with almost every bill considered by the U.S. Senate, it is unlikely that any program related to financing of long-term care for victims of HIV diseases will emerge without action on long-term care coverage in general. As noted before, it seems much easier for politicians to vote funds for research than to vote monies to assist the current group of victims.

With the pressing need to address these issues and the remote possibility that the federal government, faced with a two-trillion dollar debt, will embark on a costly new public program, is it likely that we will do anything but continue to muddle through? The pessimistic but likely answer is no. There simply is not the political constituency to force action on the problem. Even the considerable political force of the elderly has been insufficient as of now to force action on the issue of long-term care for that group. This could, however, change dramatically with the election of a less private enterprise-oriented President. More likely is the further development of joint federal-state programs other than Medicaid (such as block grants or a separate "AIDS/Medicaid-like" program) with special payments for and designation of categorical (disease-specific) providers and facilities, (e.g., New York Hospital-based AIDS treatment centers), or the use of specialized home care programs. It is likely that state and local governments will continue to play a central role in service delivery and financing (via Medicaid and special programs) since it seems easier to get political action in areas where AIDS is common.

Our look at what could be is not complete without acknowledging that current efforts to derive a more reasonable approach to long-term care for victims of HIV diseases are also hampered by the lack of an adequate data base on the distribution and use of existing services. To develop the details of a program for an effective financing and delivery system for care of those with HIV-related diseases requires information concerning comparative costs and efficacy of varying arrays and types of inpatient, outpatient, hospice, and home care services (Department of Health and Human Services 1987). Funding for research to explore these issues would appear to be vital if we are to make substantial progress.

Conclusions

It is our contention that the United States should have a means of financing long-term care for persons with HIV diseases based largely on public financing at the federal level. The eligibility should be universal, and a mix of integrated and "disease-specific" services should be provided. To develop the consensus and political action necessary to bring about such a change will be very difficult given our current biases concerning both AIDS and long-term care. It is more likely that we will continue to "muddle through" with the present nonpolicy. The failure to mount a concerted effort to develop rational public policy for the long-term care of those with HIV-related disorders has and will continue to cause needless human suffering and will waste increasingly limited healthcare dollars. We can only hope that the open debate of issues surrounding this problem will result in public action to redress this important aspect of the AIDS epidemic.

References

Andrulis, D. 1987. Hospital costs and revenues for care of AIDS patients. *Health Affairs* Winter: 111–118.

Arno, P.S. 1986. AIDS: A balancing act of resources. *Business and Health* 4: 20–21, 24.

Brandt, A.M. 1988. AIDS in historical perspective: Four lessons from the history of sexually transmitted diseases. *American Journal of Public Health* 78: 367–371.

Buchanan, R.J. 1988. State Medicaid coverage of AZT and AIDS-related policies. *American Journal of Public Health* 78: 432–436.

Department of Health and Human Services. 1987. Report of the Task Force on Long-Term Healthcare Policies. Washington, D.C.: Government Printing Office.

Faden, R.R., and N.E. Kass. 1988. Health insurance and AIDS: The status of state regulatory activity. *American Journal of Public Health* 78: 437–442.

Fauci, A.S. 1987. AIDS: Immunopathogenic mechanisms and research strategies. *Clinical Research* 34: 503–510.

Fruen, M.A. 1988. AIDS: A looming financial commitment. *Business and Health* 5: 24–27.

Gillis, W.E. 1987. Administrators take a stand on admitting AIDS patients. *Provider* 13: 33–34.

Iglehart, J.K. 1987. Financing the struggle against AIDS. *The New England Journal of Medicine* 317: 180–184.

Iglehart, J.K., J. Read, and J. Wells. 1987. The socioeconomic impact of AIDS on healthcare systems. *Health Affairs* Fall: 137–147.

Institute of Medicine, National Academy of Sciences. 1986. *Confronting AIDS—Directions for public health, healthcare, and research*. Washington, D.C.: National Academy Press.

Laudicina, S.S. 1987. Medicaid options for AIDS coverage focus on access, community care. *Business and Health* 4: 56–57.

Marlowe, R.C. 1987. The experienced talk about care delivery. *Provider* 13: 16, 18–19.

New York Times Editorial. 1988. The right fight against AIDS. 28 Feb.

Rothenberg, R., et al. 1987. Survival with the acquired immunodeficiency syndrome. *The New England Journal of Medicine* 317: 1297–1302.

Rowe, M.J., and C.C. Ryan. 1988. Comparing state-only expenditures for AIDS. *American Journal of Public Health* 78: 424–429.

Rudensky, M. 1986. Long-term care facilities awaiting decisions on AIDS reimbursement. *Modern Healthcare* 16: 15–18.

Sisk, J.E. 1987. The costs of AIDS: A review of the estimates. *Health Affairs* Summer: 5–21.

Smith, E. 1986. Testimony before the Subcommittee on Health and the Environment, U.S. House of Representatives, 5 Mar.

CHAPTER 12

The Policy Analyst's Perspective

Ruth S. Hanft

Care of human immunodeficient virus (HIV) patients reflects and refracts many public policy issues in healthcare including problems in prevention, access to acute and long-term care, financing, public and private roles, and resource allocation. Policy issues for HIV patients are similar to those for the total population, yet they are perhaps more visible and less likely to be resolved because of fear of contagion and value judgments made about the life-styles of these patients. With neither a vaccine nor a cure in sight in the near future, the issue of how much care to provide to the terminally ill—an issue also raised for the elderly—is implicit.

The cost of care for HIV is frequently raised as a problem, yet the same issue is rarely raised about care for patients with pancreatic cancer (terminal within a year), or shock trauma cases. This country has now accepted with little recent debate the higher lifetime costs of renal dialysis, transplantation, Alzheimer's disease, and neonatal intensive care and its consequences. One estimate of treatment costs for end-stage renal disease averaged $158,000 over a four-year period, about $30,000 in the terminal year (in 1984 prices) for some cancer patients who were not elderly. Compare this with estimates of total lifetime costs for the care of AIDS patients which range from $24,517 to $147,000 (Sisk 1987; Scitovsky 1988).

Before discussing the policy issues, particularly those of long-term care, this chapter will present a few examples of the similarities between the healthcare issues for HIV patients and for the general population.

141

Eligibility for Medicare for the disabled requires a 24-month waiting period after receipt of cash benefits, which occurs after a waiting period from the onset of the disability. In all, therefore, there is a 29-month waiting period. Since many HIV patients do not live that long and usually lose health insurance coverage when they can no longer work, they are part of the 35 to 37 million uninsured citizens, as are those disabled from other causes.

There is no national long-term care policy for anyone. Medicaid is the one program that finances a spectrum of long-term care services. Medicaid categorical and income eligibility varies widely among the states. Nine states still do not cover all those eligible for Supplementary Security Income. Recipients, even if they do qualify, must "spend down" income and assets to below the poverty level.

HIV Patient Characteristics

In order to design viable approaches to providing preventive, acute, or long-term care for the HIV-positive population, the characteristics of subsets of the population at risk must be considered. The HIV population currently consists of four general groups with some overlap. Each group presents similar and yet unique needs related to designing cost-effective delivery programs.

The first group is the homosexual and bisexual male population. Members of this community are likely to be regularly employed before or during the course of their illness with work-related health insurance to cover some of their costs. The responsiveness and social support structure of and for this population have been remarkable in all aspects, including prevention education, provision of care, and major changes in life-style—a true community response. The major problems are financing for those not employed, the availability of alternatives to hospital care, lack of family support for some patients, and employment discrimination.

The second group is that of the male drug users, largely a low income minority population where traditional health education and prevention approaches have not been successful. This population tends to be marginally employed or unemployed, therefore lacking employment-related health insurance even during the onset and early course of the illness. Their cultural values, recently reported at meetings, make acceptance of condoms, for example, difficult and place a severe risk on wives or sexual partners (Perales 1988). Furthermore, the social support systems developed by the homosexual community are virtually nonexistent among the drug abusers. In addition, homeless people make up an even more isolated subset of this community.

Women, although a smaller subgroup than the first two, are a growing population of HIV patients (Perales 1988). This group is composed mainly, although not exclusively, of addicts, sexual partners of addicts, and prostitutes. Reaching this population through traditional education and prevention programs poses major challenges, as do the financing of care and the development of social support systems (Perales 1988).

Finally and perhaps the saddest group is the children, who can be divided into two groups; those who have contracted the disease through blood transfusions (hopefully, a declining phenomenon) and those infected in utero (unfortunately, an increasing phenomenon). These latter infants are frequently abandoned in public hospitals (Heagarty 1988; Perales 1988). Adoption or foster care are not readily available options, and facilities other than hospitals have not been developed for care. Most nursing homes do not care for infants, nor do most home health agencies, even if a home could be found for them. Children with AIDS or AIDS-related complex (ARC) or who have tested positive for antibodies are isolated from friends, community, and schools.

The reason for discussing these demographics is to highlight some of the complexities in addressing the prevention, and acute, and long-term care delivery problems of AIDS patients. What works for the homosexual community may not work for the other subgroups just as what was designed for the elderly populations is not easily adapted to other populations.

Financing Acute HIV Care

The problems of healthcare financing are the same whether one is addressing categories of disease, age, or minority populations. The major exception is that private insurance has moved overtly to exclude individuals who test positive for the HIV antibodies. With the new genetic markers available for many latent diseases, private insurance exclusion attitudes related to HIV may be a bellwether of the future. These attitudes are a consequence of the absence of a national healthcare financing policy and of experience rating in private health and life insurance. Experience rating preexisting condition clauses requiring examinations for health insurance coverage have several consequences including:

1.   The restriction of employability of people with certain health conditions who might otherwise be able to work,

2.   An ever-growing group of uninsured and uninsurable people, and

3.   Wide variations in premium costs which provide incentives for employers to avoid hiring certain individuals.

And what of public programs? As mentioned earlier, Medicare for the disabled is not a viable option for individuals who do not live for more than two years beyond their disability onset. Furthermore, the waiting period before eligibility for Medicare encompasses the period of high cost treatment. Eligibility for HIV patients under Medicaid is subject to all the anomalies of Medicaid for other groups except that Medicaid in most states excludes single males until they are declared totally and permanently disabled.

The result of this patchwork of financing programs for the HIV patient is that in addition to the emotional impact and pain of having contracted a terminal illness, the patient becomes totally impoverished. The result for our healthcare delivery system is that an already uneven burden placed on public hospitals and clinics and certain nonprofit hospitals—notably certain teaching hospitals—is exacerbated by a new and growing group of uncompensated patients.

The issue is not HIV *per se*. The issue is an irrational healthcare financing system and an irrational incentive system that penalizes employers for hiring and retaining individuals with health problems, that rewards providers who are "profit seekers," and penalizes those who retain the primary mission of caring for the ill. Has the concept of health as a merit good been abandoned? What it ever really a goal?

The price of azidothymidine (AZT) is another issue of public concern since private health insurance policies and Medicare usually do not cover outpatient drugs (Scitovsky 1988). Again, this is not merely a problem for HIV patients; it is a problem for anyone who requires the long-term use of expensive medication such as immunosuppressive drugs, outpatient chemotherapy, etc. The AIDS financing issue is really the issue of the uninsured and the lack of a national financing program.

Long-Term Care

Just as the United States has no national financing policy for acute care, neither does it have a policy for financing long-term care. In fact, there is substantially less coverage under existing programs for long-term care services than for acute care. The problem is a generic one. However, there are more complex issues related to HIV patients since the focus of the long-term care debate has been primarily the elderly, and the system that exists now was designed for the elderly.

The definition of long-term care has been medicalized, yet it also encompasses housing, social, and personal care services for the frail elderly as well as the deinstitutionalized chronically mentally ill and chronically and terminally ill younger patient. Medicaid is the principal long-term care financing program, and again, coverage and services vary widely among the states. In the long-term care arena, however, there are service delivery problems in addition to financing problems for HIV patients.

1. Nursing homes and intermediate care facilities are geared to the care of the elderly with some space available for patients with degenerative diseases such as multiple sclerosis. AIDS patients regularly require special services, and additional precautions are necessary to protect health workers and other patients. Health workers in nursing homes as well as in hospitals need to be trained for the special problems of potential contagion and educated to understand that transmission of the disease occurs in a limited manner (Gambuti 1988).

In addition, existing facilities are not geared to the issues and problems of caring for terminally ill younger populations (Rango 1988).

2.   Home healthcare also has focused on the needs of the elderly.

3.   Addicts pose the additional special problems of detoxification and emotional disturbance.

4.   Family support is even less likely for HIV patients than for the elderly. Not only are many families unable to care for these patients because of distance and lack of caregivers, but many have rejected their homosexual sons. Prostitutes and addicts are equally or more unlikely to have family support systems which can cope with their needs.

Costs of Care

Much has been made of the high costs of caring for AIDS patients with the unstated question, "Is it worth the cost for someone who will die soon?" The following factors also need to be considered.

1.   The costs of caring for HIV patients vary widely depending on the particular manifestations of the disease, the duration of the disease, and the availability of alternatives to acute inpatient care (Scitovsky 1988).

2.   The costs of caring for an HIV patient are no higher than the costs of transplantation, many neonatal intensive care cases, shock trauma, and certain cancers where patients often do not survive for a year (Scitovsky and Rice 1987).

3.   Similarly, the costs of caring for an HIV patient are no higher than the costs of protracted degenerative illnesses such as Alzheimer's disease, multiple sclerosis, Huntington's chorea, end-stage renal disease, and schizophrenia.

The real issue is rationing—how limited resources are distributed in an equitable manner. Currently, services are rationed on the basis of the ability to pay or of one's physical access to care, not usually on the basis of the cost of illness itself (Freeman et al. 1987; Reinhardt 1987).

Ethical Issues

There are two types of ethical concerns: the generic issues of equity, justice, beneficence, and autonomy, and the specific ethical issues exemplified by HIV. This society has dealt sporadically and inconclusively with these general ethical issues. Regarding equity and justice, there has been discussion about a "right to healthcare" (undefined as to type and quantity) in the 1960s and 1970s. The President's Commission for the Study of Ethical Problems in Medicine and Biomedical and Behavioral Research (1983) introduced a concept of equitable access to adequate care without undue burdens, both of which were again undefined. Furthermore, market-oriented concepts were inadequate to explain a seriously imperfect market.

However, there are a few HIV-specific issues that merit discussion because they exemplify very hard choices, and even though they are implicit, they are rarely raised in societal decision making.

The first issue is the most visible. If the source of the transmission of the disease is known, is it the responsibility of public bodies to protect society over religious and "moral" objections? What is the public role in protecting the public good? In this instance, the public good includes dissemination of educational information, contraceptives, and perhaps even clean needles to prevent the spread of the disease. How is protection of the larger public balanced with deeply held moral beliefs? Where does the right to privacy end and the protection of others begin? It is clear that no one should knowingly spread the disease to others, but is it the right of insurers, employers, or the government to know about a specific individual who is not a danger to another individual? Is it the right of these groups to know that an individual carries the Huntington's chorea gene? Why should HIV be treated differently than any sexually transmitted disease or potential gene defect in terms of mandatory or voluntary testing?

Conclusions

In summary, although HIV may present some additional complexities in the issues and problems of financing, delivering, and rationing healthcare, the issues and problems are basically no different from financing and delivering care for a range of catastropic and high cost illnesses and even noncatastrophic illnesses. The issues are:

1.   Assuring some societally determined universal level of access to a range of health and social services,

2.   Developing national policies for defining, financing, and delivering long-term care for vulnerable citizens, whether supported through the income, housing, health, or social service programs,

3.   Protecting the public against preventable contagious diseases ranging from those which are sexually transmitted diseases to those which are spread in other ways such as measles, polio, etc., while retaining the rights of the potential patient as to confidentiality, privacy, employment, and access to public education, and

4.   Developing rational and equitable policies for rationing finite services or dollars.

While HIV is particularly visible because of ignorance, fear, homophobia, and the catastrophic effects of the illness, the issues are basically those which have been debated for years: resource allocation, access, catastrophic costs, long-term care (defining and financing), individual versus societal rights, and public and private roles in providing healthcare in the United States.

References

Freeman, H.E., et al. 1987. Americans report on their access to healthcare. *Health Affairs* 6: 6–18.

Gambuti, G. 1988. Personnel requirements: A view from the hospital. *In The AIDS patient: An action agenda. Cornell University Medical College Fourth Conference on Health Policy*, ed. D.E. Rogers and E. Ginzberg. Boulder, CO: Westview Press Inc. 50-55.

Heagarty, M.C. 1988. AIDS, IV drug use, and children. *In The AIDS Patient: An action agenda. Cornell University Medical College Fourth Conference on Health Policy,* ed. D.E. Rogers and E. Ginzberg. Boulder, CO: Westview Press Inc. 89-96.

Perales, C. 1988. Social services for people with AIDS: The state perspective. *In The AIDS patient: An action agenda. Cornell University Medical College Fourth Conference on Health Policy,* ed. D.E. Rogers and E. Ginzberg, 116–126. Boulder, CO: Westview Press Inc.

President's Commission for the Study of Ethical Problems in Medicine and Biomedical and Behavioral Research. 1983. *Securing access to healthcare.* Vol. 1. Washington, D.C.: Government Printing Office.

Rango, N. 1988. Nursing home care for people with AIDS. *In The AIDS patient: An action agenda. Cornell University Medical College Fourth Conference on Health Policy,* ed. D.E. Rogers and E. Ginzberg. Boulder, CO: Westview Press Inc. 35-41.

Reinhardt, U.E. 1987. Health insurance for the nation's poor. *Health Affairs* 6: 101–112.

Scitovsky, A.A. 1988. The economic impact of AIDS. *Health Affairs* 7: 32–45.

Scitovsky, A.A., and D. Rice. 1987. Estimates of the direct and indirect costs of acquired immunodeficiency syndrome in the United States, 1985, 1986, and 1990. *Public Health Reports* Jan.-Feb.: 5–17.

Sisk, G.E. 1987. The costs of AIDS: A review of the estimates. *Health Affairs* 6: 5–21.

CHAPTER 13

The Public Health Perspective

Reed V. Tuckson

The issues of AIDS and long-term care are of great interest to the District of Columbia's Commission of Public Health. In order not to be redundant, this chapter will concentrate on a few key elements that have not been discussed previously and that are important for the development of a long-term care system for persons with AIDS. These three elements are (1) the process by which the District of Columbia will formulate a public policy in this area; (2) the development of the models of care arrangements; and (3) the organization and management of the AIDS long-term care system.

The Public Policy Process

The formulation of a public policy in response to the multiple challenges presented to this society by the human immunodeficiency virus (HIV) epidemic is a most fascinating and important process. Given the range of uncertainties, the highly charged emotional atmosphere surrounding these issues, the moral and ethical imperatives that must be honored, and the many other competing demands for scarce resources, and finally, the manner in which we as an organized society approach decision-making assumes fundamental significance. The first steps in formulating policy direction are to understand clearly the dimension of the long-term care needs for persons with HIV disease and to define the characteristics of those needs by type of service and demography. At this point in the history of the epidemiological data base, there remains great uncertainty as to our ability to quantify or predict these variables with the precision that planners would desire. However, it is also true that there is a significant amount of good data on actual numbers of diagnosed cases of AIDS as well as descriptions of those persons. There are also useful experiential data that describe the current demand for long-term care services and that indicate areas of inadequate supply. Finally, there is knowledge of the trends in HIV prevalence and a special awareness for the implications of the increasing number of infected men and women who are either intravenous drug abusers themselves or who are their sexual partners. It is clear that many dedicated persons are part of a care system that has adequately met the needs of persons with AIDS in a responsible manner to date, that it is appropriate to reevaluate this system to better meet future demands, and that more resources will be needed for those demands.

The political process involved in the allocation of this city's scarce resources is of obvious importance. The mayor and the city council must evaluate these needs against a plethora of other pressing and expensive competing demands such as those of the criminal justice and drug abuse challenges, for example. It is important to remember that all of this discussion occurs in a context of 117,000 uninsured citizens in a city of 640,000 people, a healthcare industry that "absorbed" $100 million of uncompensated care last year, and a population that suffered 1,484 excess premature deaths last year from six chronic diseases. There are already too few resources to meet preexisting major health challenges or their long-term care implications. Now, the new burdens presented by HIV disease will certainly force some very unpleasant allocation decisions. Therefore, great clarity and responsibility are required of those committed to the education and advocacy efforts directed toward elective officials.

Models of Care Arrangements

In terms of the challenges involved in developing the elements of a continuum of care system, philosophically and economically it is preferable to house persons with AIDS in their natural home environment in a least-restrictive, most appropriate manner supplemented by an array of supportive social services. The extraordinary efforts of the District's Whitman Walker Clinic Buddy System, for example, demonstrate an extremely flexible, compassionate, and cost-effective means of providing such services. This system works because of the expertise of the clinic and the reality of a well-organized and highly motivated gay community. The new challenge will be to create such a system to serve the needs of poor and substance-abusing persons who suffer not only from multiple social support deficits but also from a lack of social organization. Although intravenous drug abusers are well organized for the distribution of narcotics, they are poorly organized for much else.

Similarly, the gay communities' initiative and support for conjugate housing services have filled the need for the next level of long-term care service. The Schwartz Housing System, also operated by the Whitman Walker Clinic, has been an exemplary public, private, and voluntary cooperative venture. At this point, the demand for this service does meet the available supply quite well. It is encouraging that other organizations have recently come forward to supply housing for other constituencies that have not been targeted previously. The Damien Ministries, a local religious movement, has been critical in addressing the needs of women and substance abusers. Nevertheless, more will be required to meet the conjugate housing needs of the ever-increasing poor and substance-abusing HIV-infected population. The difficulty, as always, is financing. The Schwartz Housing System benefited greatly from the fund-raising activities of the gay and lesbian community. The new demand can be expected to fall almost exclusively on the resources of the city.

As this long-term care system evolves, the need for a new type of housing arrangement is becoming evident. This more medically intensive housing should serve as a cost-effective intermediate point between the traditional conjugate house and the hospital. An array of medical interventions, including the use of intravenous therapy, would be possible in this setting. These homes would serve as part of the continuum both before and after hospitalization. More work needs to be devoted to the design and management of such facilities, but the idea seems to have merit.

Moving along the continuum of care, the District has been able, through the use of government facilities, to meet the nursing home needs of persons with AIDS. However, as future requirements unfold, the private sector nursing home community will have to shoulder its fair share of the burden. Training efforts are currently in progress to help dispel the fears and anxieties of the staff members at such facilities as one effort to reduce the barriers to private sector involvement. Certainly, public sector health insurance funding will be increasingly required to finance this need. At this time there is not as clear a sense as would be desired of the ultimate need for nursing home placements for persons with AIDS over the next few years. Planning efforts will have to address this uncertainty.

Regarding hospice care, local inpatient hospice needs in this area have been well met by the Washington Home, which is in the process of expanding, and to date, has matched the demands placed on it. Expanding the availability of in-home hospice care is of current interest. As discussed earlier, the Washington area is increasing its ability to provide the full array of supportive services to home-bound persons with AIDS. These efforts also permit the provision of cost-effective, least restrictive, most appropriate, in-home hospice care as well. The efforts of Hospice Care of the District of Columbia, the only accredited outpatient hospice program in the area, deserves recognition in this effort.

Finally, special emphasis should be given to the needs of the unfortunately large and growing population of babies with HIV diseases. Washington, D.C. is trying to avoid the "boarder baby" syndrome that has frustrated hospitals in New York City. Babies with AIDS are born to women who have their own plethora of needs and deficits. Often they will be unable to care either for themselves or their babies. It is inappropriate morally, socially, and economically for such babies to live in hospitals. Unfortunately, there has always been inadequate foster care and adoptive resources for minority babies.

The District is indeed fortunate to have Grandma's House available to its HIV-infected children. This marvelous house —a model where the mother and the baby can be housed together and which permits the mother to be involved with the care of her child as she herself receives the support necessary to function—was created by two caring and sensitive black women and is supported by a mixture of public and private money. The babies are cared for with love and compassion, and the House is a true beacon of light and hope for the future. Although at present, the available facilities have met the needs, unquestionably more such facilities will be required in the near future.

Organization and Management

The third and final element of this discussion is the need to develop a management structure which permits and facilitates the movement of people through the continuum of care system. The foundation of such a system is a case management ability that assesses individual needs, coordinates the available resources, arranges the financing, and tracks the person as needs and services change. It is necessary to decide who these case managers will be, how they will be compensated, and for whom they will work. For example, the District government now operates several systems of case management for persons in many different need categories. Should the existing systems be redefined to accommodate persons with AIDS? Should a new system be created specifically to address the concerns of those persons? What should the relationship be between the government and the staffs of the private sector resource suppliers? Should the District let the private sector providers work out these relationships among themselves without centralized local government involvement, as occurs in San Francisco? Do the special needs of increasing numbers of poor persons with multiple preexisting deficits necessitate a more vigorous centralized governmental registry and tracking system?

These are difficult questions which are presently under analysis. Certainly financial and labor resource variables will shape the final decisions. However, the goal of the D.C. Commission of Public Health is to achieve a management system that is efficient, flexible, and best at meeting responsibilities to the client.

Conclusions

As with all other aspects of the fight against the HIV epidemic, communities must remain united and true to the highest ideals of our civilization. As the difficult resource allocation decisions are made, the goal should be to prevent an "us against them" mentality. In developing community placements for persons with AIDS, selfishness and ignorant discrimination should not impede their acceptance and establishment.

So far there has been some success in working together to meet the long-term care needs of several cities' HIV-infected population. As there is further progress in the medical treatment of this disease, as infected persons live longer and require more care, and as there are more persons who will place themselves at risk because of their inappropriate behavior, these care needs will only increase. How local communities prepare to address the future will describe what kind of a people we are.

CHAPTER 14

The Federal Perspective

Robert E. Windom

It is impossible, or at best unproductive to consider the long-term care of the AIDS patient without examining a few salient facets of the AIDS epidemic itself. It is known, for example, that the epidemic is still expanding, both in real numbers and in geographic dispersion. What this expansion should indicate is that health professionals *generally*, not just those who practice in certain cities or regions of the country, must be alerted to the spread of the disease and given educational assistance in its diagnosis and treatment.

Twenty-one percent of the AIDS cases reported to date have been diagnosed in New York City, and about another 8% have occurred in both San Francisco and Los Angeles. Cases have tended to cluster in urban areas, and some cities have been far harder hit than others. AIDS has surfaced, however, in every state and territory, and no matter where a health professional practices, he or she can expect to see cases of AIDS before very long.

It is also known that the human immunodeficiency virus (HIV) is found in many types of body fluids and is spread from infected persons to those who are not infected by certain specific behaviors.

It is obvious that health professionals who have drug abusers or homosexual men as patients ought to know as much as possible about AIDS and how it is diagnosed and treated, but *any* practitioner may have a patient, male or female, who has been infected by HIV because of an encounter with an infected person, transfusion of an infectious unit of blood before screening, or hemophilia. An understanding of the modes of transmission can be a valuable diagnostic tool.

Although the overwhelming majority of AIDS patients have been adults, a small, but growing, minority have been children, especially the newborns of intravenous drug abusers. Another important aspect of the disease is that while it has spread mainly among white adult males, a sizable and growing proportion of the total number of persons with AIDS are young blacks and Hispanics.

It is clear that when considering AIDS or, more to the point, people who are infected with HIV, it is necessary to put aside fixed generalizations about the disease or the people infected. They do not always apply. This is especially important when considering the impact that the AIDS epidemic can be expected to have on patient care in general (on facilities and personnel) and on long-term care in particular.

Intragovernmental Task Force on AIDS Healthcare Delivery

In January 1987, Dr. David Sundwall, Administrator of Health Resources and Services Administration, was requested to call a top level interagency intradepartmental task force to look at all of the issues related to the delivery of healthcare to persons infected by HIV.

Dr. Sundwall brought together experts from the Departments of Defense, State, Housing and Urban Development, Health and Human Services, and the Veterans Administration. They met throughout last year, and examined the issues set before them.

In general, the task force found no problems with the way acute care has been provided to AIDS patients. The system is far from perfect, of course, but it has been doing a commendable job given the size of the task, the diversity of our society, and the numbers of people served. The task force found that our healthcare system has responded appropriately to the AIDS crisis by making available a wide range of services.

The report did, however, identify some gaps in the present state of healthcare delivery, and some of these gaps are especially relevant to long-term care. Using these gaps as their basis of discussion, the task force offered 17 recommendations covering a broad spectrum of issues including access to care, quality of care, and financing.

The first recommendation concerns health professionals. The task force said that something needs to be done to ". . . improve the education of health professionals in the diagnosis, care, and counseling of HIV-infected individuals" (U.S. Department of Health and Human Services 1988). In other words, healthcare professionals *anywhere* who are involved in providing some aspect of healthcare to people with AIDS need to know much more about the disease than they may have picked up from reading their professional journals, from their continuing education courses, or from newspapers and television. They need to know, for example

1. much more than most do now about the high risk behaviors that lead to AIDS;

2. the cultural, racial, and ethnic composition of the people who have had AIDS so far;

3. more about the growing number of really difficult ethical and legal issues that keep occurring;

4. more about case management techniques and interdisciplinary teamwork; and

5. a great deal more about the epidemiology and prevention of those high risk behaviors that lead to AIDS.

These are the kinds of topics and issues that should be incorporated into any educational plan or program for health professionals who provide care for persons infected with the HIV. The Public Health Service has funded four AIDS regional education and training centers to begin to address these problems. The Department of Health and Human Services intends to increase that number in 1989. Excellent work in this area has already begun by the American Medical Association, the American Hospital Association, the American Nurses Association, and many other professional groups.

The task force also recommended that the government provide AIDS-related education and training for personnel in federally funded healthcare projects such as community health and drug abuse treatment centers. It also recommended that the Department of Health and Human Services review all of its programs and policies to make sure that the confidentiality of AIDS patients is protected to the fullest possible extent. In a related recommendation, the task force urged the Department of Health and Human Services to explore ways in which it might act to protect persons with AIDS from acts of discrimination.

With regard to long-term care specifically, the task force recommended that the supply of intermediate and long-term care facilities be expanded to provide more in-patient care for AIDS patients. This expansion, the task force suggested, should be carried out under the terms of Section 232 of the National Housing Act, which authorizes FHA mortgage loan guarantees for the construction of skilled nursing facilities.

The Department will be looking at this recommendation to see how it might be implemented jointly by the Department of Health and Human Services (DHHS) and the Department of Housing and Urban Development (HUD). Congress has provided $6.7 million for limited construction during fiscal year 1988.

The task force concluded that the burden of caring for AIDS patients has been carried to a disproportionate extent by general acute care hospitals. What is lacking is a supply of nonhospital-based, nonacute care intermediate and long-term care facilities that would absorb much of the present patient load and, probably, most of the AIDS patients in the future.

These kinds of facilities are needed, but the nursing home industry does not seem inclined to generate them on its own. The task force members therefore suggested that the Department of Health and Human Services try to discover the reasons for this reluctance as soon as possible.

Meanwhile, the task force recommended that the government take steps to encourage medical day care and foster care for adult and pediatric AIDS patients. For many AIDS patients, these would be acceptable and appropriate alternatives to in-patient institutional care. Day care and foster care are state-controlled activities, of course, but the federal government should have a role in encouraging their use for AIDS patients and in generating information about these approaches to care and how and where they should be employed.

Conclusions

Last year, our nation's healthcare system took care of tens of thousands of AIDS patients at an estimated total cost of well over one billion dollars. It has been estimated, however, that in a few years, approximately 172,000 people will have symptoms of AIDS or AIDS-related diseases and will require medical assistance. Some experts have projected the cost of providing this care to be as high as $13 billion (Public Health Service 1988). Hopefully the long-term care industry will begin to work with the federal government so that a joint plan can be developed with a genuinely realistic approach to this problem of caring for the rapidly growing population of persons with AIDS.

AIDS-related activities will remain a top priority of the Public Health Service and the Department of Health and Human Services for the foreseeable future. Continued research for drugs and vaccines will lead the effort. Yet dissemination of information and education to the public will be most important to control the disease in the meantime. The further spread of the virus causing this disease can be stopped in its tracks—if only individuals alter their behavior if they are at risk. Finally, with the commitment of the government, from the federal to the local level, along with increasing private and general public support, the provision for care of HIV-infected persons will be accomplished.

References

Public Health Service. 1988. Report of the Second Public Health Service AIDS Prevention and Control Conference—Executive summary. *Public Health Reports* 103 (Suppl. 1): 3–9.

U.S. Department of Health and Human Services. Office of Human Development Services, Health Resources Administration. 1988. *Report of the Intragovernmental Task Force on AIDS Healthcare Delivery*. GPO 1988-201-851-60434. Washington, D.C.: Government Printing Office.

```
─────────── E P I L O G U E ───────────

              A Call for Action


        Donna Lind Infeld and Richard McK. F. Southby
```

The previous chapters in this book describe the current state of health care delivery and financing for the care of AIDS patients. When the service settings discussed are merged into one comprehensive list, a continuum of care much like that developed for the elderly long-term care population can be produced.

Figure E-1 presents a compilation of several lists showing the services which make up the long-term care continuum. While this is an *ideal* listing, not reflecting real service availability, it does convey the range of options potentially available to provide long-term care services. The left column indicates services which have been used for traditional long-term care populations. The right column indicates those that are available in a few model AIDS programs or that have been identified as potentially appropriate for AIDS patients.

For each service in the continuum, specific issues need to be addressed when considering the provision of care to patients with AIDS.

Nursing Homes

Although nursing homes may be able to provide more cost-effective services for some AIDS patients than hospitals, few have been willing to accept AIDS or AIDS-related complex (ARC) patients on a routine basis. Some of the reasons for concern have been discussed throughout this book.

There are also some arguments however, *for* nursing homes to accept AIDS patients. In most situations, AIDS patients can participate in general activities without posing any danger to others.

Figure E-1 Continuum of Care Settings.

	Geriatric Long-Term Care	AIDS Long-Term Care
Institutional/Residential Environments		
Mental hospitals	X	
Acute care general hospitals	X	X
Subacute care unit	X	X
Chronic care (specialty) hospitals	X	?[a]
Rehabilitation hospitals	X	
Skilled nursing facilities	X	X
Intermediate care facilities	X	X
Congregate housing	X	X
Group home	X	X
Personal care/board and care	X	X
Foster homes	X	X
Domiciliary homes	X	?
Retirement homes	X	
Hospice care	X	X
Respite care	X	X
Community-Based		
Hospice care	X	X
Respite care	X	X
Outpatient clinics	X	X
Adult day care: medical model	X	X
Adult day care: social model	X	?
Recreation programs	X	X
Mental health care	X	X
Spiritual services	X	X
Sheltered workshops	X	?
Dental services	X	X
Community medical services	X	X
Senior centers	X	
Legal/protective services	X	X
Nutrition programs/congregate meals	X	
Transportation programs	X	X
Home-Based		
Home health care/nursing and therapies	X	X
Meals on wheels	X	X
Nurse aide/attendant care	X	X
Homemaker	X	X
Chore service	X	X
Medical monitoring services	X	X
Home repair and handyman services	X	X
Friendly visitors	X	X
Telephone reassurance	X	X

[a] ? means that these services are not currently available for AIDS patients, have not been discussed in the literature, but may be worthy of consideration.

Figure E-1, continued.

	Geriatric Long-Term Care	AIDS Long-Term Care
Coordination		
Discharge planning	X	X
Assessment	X	X
Case management/service management	X	X
Information and referral	X	X
Income maintenance/entitlement education	X	X
Training of caregivers and volunteers	X	X

Providers also have a moral obligation to care for anyone who needs services. Administrators may consider that if nursing homes do not accept AIDS patients, then hospitals might become licensed to provide long-term care. Finally, some states are providing financial incentives to facilities which admit AIDS patients. Each of the settings in the continuum of care should carefully examine both sides of the issue of providing AIDS care.

Issues and Questions for Consideration

Looking at the question of whether AIDS patients should be served in the existing long-term care service settings or in separate specialty settings is part of the issue to which there seems to be a growing consensus. The opinions expressed throughout this book suggest that existing long-term care settings have a role, a responsibility, and a reason to provide care to AIDS patients. While separate wings or units are often appropriate, separate organizations or institutions are generally not. Even when specialty settings are perceived to be preferable (when there are special services provided that are not available in other settings), their creation is generally not realistic. This is especially true in low incidence areas.

Thus, the challenge becomes more difficult. Who can be served most effectively in which settings and how can we be sure that those services are available? Specific questions which emerged throughout the book and which need further attention include the following.

1.   How can care for AIDS patients be organized into a system which includes coordinated care, social services, and cost-effective managed care arrangements?

2.   How can programs be organized to provide appropriate care in low, moderate, and high incidence areas?

3.   Will new AIDS services reduce funds available to support geriatric long-term care?

4.   What are the roles of specific long-term care facilities and services for various disease manifestations and different high risk populations?

5.   How will the inclusion of AIDS patients affect staffing of long-term care programs?

6.   Will new programs result in inefficiencies and redundancies of services?

7.   Will a separate service system further stereotype and stigmatize AIDS patients?

8.   How can research on these service delivery questions be encouraged?

9.   What policy changes at the federal, state, and local levels are needed to address these problems?

These are not easy questions. While there are little data available to answer them, at least they are being asked. If this book has begun to clarify them, it will have met its goal. If it stimulates further research and influences policy agendas, it will have made an important contribution to meeting the needs of all patients who need long-term care.

Access, xxii, 123
Acute care, 156
Adult day care, xxi
Advisory panel, 129-130
AIDS
    attitudes, on homosexuality, 38
    cases reported, 6
    changes in clinical manifestations, 53
    defined, xviii
    demographics, 155-156
    emotional aspects, 24
    epidemiology, 6-7
    episodic nature, 84
    geographic spread, 155
    as handicap, 90
    historical perspective, 3-4
    incubation period, 5
    latency time, 32-33
    natural history, 5-6
    population, changes, 53
    psychological symptoms, 32
    psychological terror, 30
    as stigmatizing disease, 30
AIDS long-term care system, 50-55
    case management, 52
    community attitude, 54
    community organizations, 52
    development, 53-54
        new treatment protocols, 53
    financing, 54
    objectives, 50
    obstacles, 55
    provider organizations, 52
    public support, 54
    resource availability, 54
    system components, 50-52
        assessment, 50
        early intervention, 51
        education, 50
        inpatient hospital care, 51

    nonacute organized healthcare, 51
    outpatient hospital care, 51
    prevention, 50
    residential care, 51-52
AIDS patient care network, 122-123
AIDS Project Los Angeles, 106
AIDS-related complex (ARC), xvii
AIDS unit, 61, 94
Anger, 32
Anticipatory grief, 40
Antidiscrimination law, 90
Anxiety, 30-31, 32
ARC, xvii
Assessment, 50
Autonomy, 35, 145
    long-term care, 82
    nursing home, 82
Azidothymidine (AZT)
    cost, 143
    Medicaid, 118

Beneficence, 35, 145
Biomedical research, 129
Blood exposure
    prevention, 15
    risk, 15
Boarder baby, 141, 152
Burnout, 94

Cancer, 31
    psychological reactions, 31-32
        prognosis, 31
Care model, 150-153
Care setting, continuum, 162-163
Case management, xxi, 52, 153
Casual transmission, 9
Catastrophic protection, 102
Centers for Disease Control recommendations, 16, 91
    cost, 93
    rationale, 16
Charity, 104-105
Child with AIDS, xxiii, 141, 152-153

Cognitive deficit, 108. *See also* Dementia
Communicable disease law, 89-91
Community attitude, AIDS long-term care system, 54
Community-based services, xxi
Community hospital, 23
Community involvement
     long-term care, 83
     nursing home, 83
Community organization, 52
Confidentiality, 33, 34
     doctor-patient communication, 34
Congregate living setting, 85
Conjugate housing service, 151
Cost, xxii, 101-107, 109-110, 130, 139, 144-145. *See also*
     Reimbursement
     acute care, 141-143
     azidothymidine, 143
     CDC guidelines, 93
     financing patterns, 104-107
     long-term care, 143-144
     nursing home, 64-65
     state role, 113-123, 130
     uncompensated care, 105
     vs. other diseases, 139
Cost study protocol, 106
Criminalization, 33-34
Cryptococcal meningitis, 6
Cytomegalovirus, 6

Damien Ministries, 151
Day care, 158
Death, hospice, 70, 72
Dementia, 25, 26, 27, 108
     home care, 84-85
     hospice, 73-74
Dental professional, HIV incidence, 15
Deontological theory, 34-36
Depression, 24, 30-31, 32
Discharge appeals process, 91
Discharge disposition, 48, 49
Discharge to home, 48, 49
Disease-specific program, 122

District of Columbia's Commission of Public Health, 149-154
    care models, 150-153
    management, 153
    public policy process, 149-150
Do not resuscitate policy, nursing home, 84
Doctor-patient communication, confidentiality, 34
Drug user, xxiv, 140-141
    nursing home, 78

Early intervention, 51
Education, 50, 92, 94
    healthcare worker, 157-158
    materials, 59
    nursing home, 58
Educational materials, nursing home, 58-60
Emergency room, 24
Enzyme-linked immunosorbent assay (ELISA), 4
Equity, 145
Ethical issues, 33-36, 91-92, 145
    education, 92, 94
    family, 94-95
    lover, 95
    provision of care, 91-92
Ethnic group, 7

Family, 23, 26
    ethical issues, 94-95
    grief, 40-41
    hospice, 27
    informal care, 108
    of origin, 40-41
Fear, 29
Female AIDS patient, 141
Financial case management, 105
Financing, AIDS long-term care system, 54
Foster care, 158
Funding, 37

Gay community, 29, 41, 151
Gay-lesbian community, 132
Gay male, xxiii, 140
    expressing feelings, 40

psychosocial issues, 29-42
Gene amplification, 5
Grandma's House, 152-153
Grief, 29, 39-41
  anticipatory, 40
  family, 40-41
Group health insurance, continued coverage, 103, 117, 132
Guilt, 32

Health insurance risk pool, 116
Health Resources and Services Administration AIDS service delivery
    demonstration program, 106
Heathcare worker
  anxiety, 3
  blood exposure, 10
  education, 157-158
    nursing home, 58
  homophobia, 38-39
  insensitivity, 26
  no identifiable risk behavior, 10
  prospective longitudinal studies, 12-16
  risk, 9-16
    epidemiology, 9-10
  seroconversion, 11-12
Helping network, 40
Hepatitis
  effects, 14
  healthcare worker risk, 14
  risk for transmission, 14
Hepatitis B vaccine, 8-9
HIV, 4
  blood test, 4
  casual transmission, 9
  defined, xviii
  historical perspective, 3-4
  natural history, 5-6
  occupational risk, 9-16
  pathogenesis, 4-5
  patient characteristics, 140-141
  prevalence, 17
  prevention, 16-19
  serological tests, 4-5

status consequences, 32
    virus, 4-5
HIV-1. *See* HIV
HIV-positive patient, mainstreaming, 61
HIV-related disorder, xviii
Home care, xxi, 84-85, 150-151
    dementia, 84-85
    Medicaid, 119-121
    reimbursement, 85
Homophobia, 32, 37-39
    defined, 38
    healthcare worker, 38-39
    internalized, 38
Hospice, xxi, 69-76, 152
    AIDS care implementation, 73-75
    care site, 70
    caregiver support, 74-75
    commitment, 71-73
    concept, 70-71
    death, 70, 72
    dementia, 73-74
    family, 27
    level of care, 73-74
    multidisciplinary team, 71
    provider concerns, 75
    psychosocial needs, 74
    spiritual needs, 74
    staff education, 71-73
        AIDS transmissibility, 72
        confronting death, 72
        patient population, 73
    symptom management, 73-74
Hospice Care of the District of Columbia, 152
Hospice of Washington, 69-76
    program description, 69-70
Hospital, 130
Household contact, 9
Housing, 108-109
    pediatric AIDS, 109

Immune globulin preparation, 8-9
Indigent care program, 121-122

Infective waste, 62
Informal care, 108
Informing partner, 34-36
Inpatient hospital care, 48, 51
Insurance, 66, 101-107, 130. *See also* Private insurance
    financing patterns, 104-107
    lack of coverage, 113, 114-115
    publicly financed, 133-134
        means-tested, 134
        state vs. federal, 134
Intermediate care facility, expanded supply, 158
Internalized homophobia, 38
Intragovernmental Task Force on AIDS Healthcare Delivery, 156-158
Intravenous drug user, xxiv, 140-141
    nursing home, 78
Isolation, 32
    long-term care, 81
    nursing home, 81

Justice, 145

Kaposi's sarcoma, 5

Legal issues, 33-34, 89-91, 95
Life expectancy, 107-108
Life-style, nursing home conflicts, 78
Lifelink, 41
Long-term care, 156-158
    activities program, 83
    autonomy, 82
    community involvement, 83
    cost, 143-144
    definitions, xviii
    developmentally disabled, xix
    elderly, xix
    infants, xix
    isolation, 81
    placement needs, 80
      medical appropriateness, 80-81
    population, xix
    reimbursement, 143-144
    resource limitations, 93

service systems, xix-xxii
Long-term care facility, expanded supply, 158
Long-term care insurance, 133
Loss, 39-41
Lover
    ethical issues, 95
    informing, 34-36

Mainstreaming, 110, 134, 163
Medicaid, xxiii, 90, 91, 101-107, 130-131
    1987 AIDS cost, 117
    AIDS cost percentage, 117
    AIDS coverage, 118
    azidothymidine, 118
    disability, 131
    financing patterns, 104-107
    home care, 119-121
    state role, 117-121
    waiting period, 103
Medical day care, 158
Medicare, 90, 91, 142
    disability, 103, 114
    reimbursement
        home care, 102
        hospice, 102
Mind-body unity concept, 31-32
Mycobacterium avium-intracellulare, 5-6, 26, 27-28

NAPH/COTH study, 48-49
National Association of People with AIDS, 41
National Center for Health Services Research, 106
Needlestick, 11, 62
Neurological disorder, xxiv, 24
No identifiable risk behavior, 7
    healthcare worker, 10
Nonacute organized healthcare, 51
Nonmaleficence, 35
Nursing home, 57-67, 151-152, 158, 161-163
    activities program, 83
    adjustments, 70
    aggressive treatment, 83

AIDS patients access, 119
AIDS patients refusal, 57
autonomy, 82
barriers, 77-79
care guidelines, 78-79
care intensity, 79
characterized, xx
community involvement, 83
dental services, 63-64
do not resuscitate policy, 84
education, 58
educational materials, 58-60
episodic care, 84
experimental drug, 63
HIV-positive employee, 66-67
infection control, 78
initial staff education, 58
isolation, 81
IV drug abuser, 78
life-style conflicts, 78
managerial concerns, 61-67
    cost, 64-65
    facility competence, 61-64
    media exposure, 65
    workers' compensation, 65-67
palliative care, 83-84
patient concerns, 60-61
    AIDS unit, 61
    mainstreaming, 61
    reassurance, 60-61
physician services, 63
placement need, 80
    medical appropriateness, 80-81
quality incentive payments, 119
reimbursement, 79
resource limitations, 93
staff concerns, 58-60
staff education, 78-79
staff family concerns, 58-60
traditional role, 81-83
Universal Precautions, 62

Occupational Safety and Health Administration, 18-19, 91
    employee precautions, 18-19
    enforcement, 19
Out-of-hospital placement, 48
Outpatient hospital care, 51

Pain, 27
Palliative care, 80-81
    nursing home, 83-84
Patient family concerns, 60-61
    AIDS unit, 61
    mainstreaming, 61
    reassurance, 60-61
Patient population, 128
    patient characteristics, 140-141
Pneumocystis carinii pneumonia, 3, 5
Policy, lack of, 36-37
Preoccupation with illness, 32
Prevention, 50
    policy issues, 145
Private insurance, 110-111, 131-132
    screening, 132, 141-142
    state incentive, 116-117
Private insurer, screening, 114, 115-116
    legislation restricting, 115
Prospective cost study, 106-107
Prospective study, healthcare worker risk, 12-16
Provider organization, 52
Provision of care, 91-92
Provision of service, 90-91
Psychiatric institution, 25
Psychological disorder, 24
Psychological support, 94
Psychosocial issues, 29-42
Psychosocial needs, hospice, 74
Public Health Service recommendations, 16
    rationale, 16-17
Public hospital, 130
Public policy, 129
    process, 149-150
Public support, AIDS long-term care system, 54

Quality of care, xxii

Race, 7
Rationing, 145
Reimbursement, xxiii, 101-107. *See also* Cost
    acute care, 141-143
    financing patterns, 104-107
    home care, 85
    long-term care, 143-144
    Medicare
        home care, 102
        hospice, 102
        nursing home, 79
        outside hospital, 55
Repeat testing, 5
Research, 129
Residential care, xx, 51-52, 109
Respite care, xxi
Retrovirus, 4-5
Right to health care, 103-104, 145
Risk pool, 116
Robert Wood Johnson Foundation demonstration project, 106

Satellite culture, 38
School Board of Nassau County v. Arline, 89-90
Schwartz Housing System, 151
Screening, 95
    private insurer, 114, 115-116, 132, 141-142
        legislation restricting, 115
Segregation, 134, 163
Self-governance, 35
Self-help group, 40
Self-image, 30
Seroconversion
    healthcare worker, 11-12
    rate per event, 12, 13
Seroconversion time, 5
Service management, xxii
Skilled nursing facility, xx
Social oppression, 37-38
Specialization, 110

Spiritual needs, hospice, 74
Staff
   contracting AIDS, 95
   education, nursing home, 58
   HIV-positive, 95
   needlestick, 95
Stigmatization, 37, 110
Stress, 30-31
   hospice staff, 74-75
Survival time, 107-108

Target population program, 122-123
Task force, 129-130
Teaching hospital, 24
Toxoplasmosis, 5
Training, Universal Precautions, 18
Transfusion recipient, 7, 23
Transmission, 128
Transmission route, 8-9

Uninsured patient, 113, 114-115, 140
Universal Precautions, 16-19, 91
   nursing home, 62
   rationale, 16-17
   training, 18
Utilitarianism, 34-36

Veterans Administration, 105
Victim blaming, 36
Volunteer, 108, 132

Washington Home, 152
Western blot, 4
Whitman Walker Clinic Buddy System, 151
Workers' compensation, 65-67
   employee testing, 66
   hiring HIV-positive employee, 66-67
   insurance, 66
   patient testing, 66